# The
# Bircher-Benner
# Health Guide

by Ruth Kunz-Bircher

*Director, the Bircher-Benner Clinic*
*Zurich, Switzerland*

*Translated from the French*
*by Rosemary Sheed*

*Published by*
Woodbridge Press Publishing Company
Santa Barbara, California

*Published and distributed by*

Woodbridge Press Publishing Company
Post Office Box 6189
Santa Barbara, California 93111

*Copyright © 1980 by Woodbridge Press Publishing Company*

English translation copyright © 1980
by George Allen & Unwin (Publishers) Ltd. London.

Originally published in French under the title
*Le Guide de Santé Bircher* © Editions Stock/Opera Mundi 1977

*Library of Congress Cataloging in Publication Data*

Kunz-Bircher, Ruth, 1902–
  The Bircher-Benner health guide.

  Translation of Le guide de santé Bircher.
  Bibliography: p.
  1. Diet therapy.  2.  Naturopathy.  3.  Zürich.
Privat–Klinik Bircher-Benner.  I.  Title.
[DNLM:  1.  Diet therapy – Popular works.  WB400
K953g]
RM216.K85513  1980      613.2′6      80-23644
ISBN 0-912800-87-9

Please note: *The health information in this book is of a general nature and is not intended to be a prescription for any specific person or condition. The application of general information such as this to a specific case should be with the counsel and guidance of a qualified health practitioner.*

# Contents

*(Measurements: Please note that both metric and English measurements are given and that
an English pint contains 20 ounces rather than 16 as in American measurements.)*

'Born to health, man spends his time undermining his heritage.'

Dr Max Bircher-Benner

The Publishers wish to thank Jacqueline Dineen and Dr Elizabeth Evans for their help in preparing the English language version of this book.

# Foreword

I have written this book about my father's life work in order to introduce to a wider public the general ideas on nutrition and their practical application in the healing of many disorders worked out in theory and in practice by the late Dr Max Bircher-Benner.

A few years after his death in 1939, I took over the administrative direction of his clinic, being already thoroughly familiar with his general objectives and the basic nutritional rules he insisted upon in his medical treatment.

During the thirty or so years of my work I had of course every opportunity to observe closely the results of my father's principles of therapy when put into practice.

The Privat-Klinik Dr Bircher-Benner, Zurich, continues today, 75 years after it was first started by Dr Max Bircher-Benner to be conducted in his spirit. His methods and therapies are practised almost without change by doctors of renown, who continue to have the same success that the founder did.

As a result of the work done at the Bircher-Benner-Klinik, various medical schools of thought have had to revise their contention that because of its greater amount of ballast, raw food is deleterious for a sick person. Today the most conventional medical journals confirm the importance that food should contain a substantial amount of fibre.

Official medical science in the past few decades has adopted many of the principles of the nutritional therapy of Dr Max Bircher-Benner, thus bringing solid proof of the correctness of his views, details of which are given in this book.

I want to thank my brothers, the late Dr Willy Bircher,

11

Dr Ralph Bircher, my cousin Dr Dagmar Liechti von Brasch, my husband Dr Alfred Kunz and all the other devoted collaborators who over the past thirty years have helped me in my work at the Bircher-Benner-Klinic.

I owe further thanks to my husband for his invaluable advice and assistance with the specifically scientific references in this book.

I also wish to express my appreciation to Mrs Margrit Michel-Muszynski for her help in preparing the manuscript.

To the publishers, Messrs George Allen & Unwin, and more particularly to Mr Peter Leek, I express my special appreciation for the careful attention and the sense of responsibility with which they have approached the production of this English language edition, and also my appreciation to Rosemary Sheed for the excellent translation.

Last but not least my appreciative thanks go to Madame M. Routier in Paris for her inspiring encouragement to produce the first version of this book in French.

*Ruth Kunz-Bircher*

# 1. The Secrets of Health

Pollution today threatens all of us. The fish die in our poisoned rivers, and even the ocean beds are turning into rubbish dumps littered with concrete containers full of indestructible radioactive waste. We stuff our land with chemical fertilisers to force it to produce more; we spray our fruit trees with pesticides we know to be poisonous. The human race is suffering from the oil civilisation, a self-inflicted sickness.

In our hyper-industrialised society, our food – from babyhood – has become a kind of Trojan horse that brings the enemy right into our midst. The few life-giving elements that remain in vegetables, fruit, dairy products, cereals, meat and fish are being destroyed by colourings and chemical preservatives. Sterilisers and antibacterial chemicals not only kill microbes; they also prevent the development of indispensable antibodies, and attack the intestinal flora. Our food thus loses its vital principles, and our capacity for self-defence is reduced, leaving us unprotected against disease. Our vulnerability is further increased by the stress of modern urban living.

What sort of help is available? What is being done to safeguard what nothing can replace – our health?

Apart from a few immunisations, there is virtually no preventive medicine today. Even family doctors now tend to practise emergency medicine only. Of course, when the city is invaded everything must be done to drive the invader out. But even when he has gone, the city will still bear the scars, and the next aggressor will find the same way in. Sometimes, too, the invader can be defeated only by destroying a building, or even a whole district, by lighting a counter-fire – and such drastic mutilation will be irreparable. But surely it would be preferable to face the

13

attacker with a strong city that can defend itself in the first place?

Everyone is aware of the danger: governments, scientists, ecologists are all wrestling with the problem of how to feed people without impoverishing the food or polluting the environment. Yet up to now no one seems to have found any world-wide solution for the immediate future. Intensive cultivation with fertilisers continues.

At the individual level, however, there is a solution that anyone can apply. It was arrived at over seventy years ago by Dr Max Bircher-Benner, though he knew nothing of the pollution we face today. He discovered and perfected a dietetic system of prevention and cure which has proved an excellent defence. It is highly relevant today.

In his early days as a young doctor, he came to realise that the only weapon the body could offer against all assaults was good health. It was to this end that he directed his research, and for over fifty years he conducted experiments both in hospital and in the clinic he founded outside Zurich. All the ingredients of his therapeutic method came from nature – air, water, sun, vegetables, fruit, cereals, dairy produce – and with these he achieved remarkable cures.

His dietetic principles are designed to prevent and to cure various illnesses, including those major killers of our day, arterial disease and certain cancers. But his dietary system must not be isolated from other aids – hydrotherapy, sun and air – nor, more important, from its philosophical framework. Bircher-Benner's method teaches not merely a new way of eating, but a new art of living. His rules of living and eating and his principles of health are easy to observe, and flexible enough to be followed when travelling as well as at home. Anyone who cannot face a total change of lifestyle can at least undertake a preventive 'detoxication' cure (see p. 127): start with an eight-day strict treatment, repeat it whenever the season changes, and add a day or two of dieting as often as possible in between. Anyone who is actually ill is advised to undertake the initial strict treatment only under the supervision of a doctor, but for such problems as obesity you can follow it on your own.

Obviously, the more closely you follow the routines stipulated, the better the results will be, but even more crucial is the choice of products to be eaten (see p. 80, on choosing and preparing fruit and vegetables). Properly followed, the Bircher-Benner dietary system is the best guard against illness, and also offers a good chance of living happily into old age without the infirmities usually associated with it.

# 2. The Beginnings

One day in January 1900 a young doctor called Max Bircher-Benner sat down after speaking for over an hour to the Medical Society of Zurich on the secrets of nutrition. The president rose to his feet:

'Monsieur Bircher has stepped beyond the bounds of science,' he said.

It was not just a verdict – it was an excommunication. Bircher was not to be allowed to continue his experiments under medical supervision at the university, as he had requested, and he could no longer be received at any medical congress or take part in any study group. A pariah at thirty-three!

As he gathered up his lecture notes before leaving, he heard the angry comments: he didn't know what he was talking about, he was bringing medicine into disrepute, his theories were dangerous nonsense. With righteous looks on their faces, his colleagues rejected him, one and all. Some clearly thought he was out of his mind.

In fact, Dr Max Bircher-Benner was a precursor of the science of nutrition (now called dietetics). At a time when the accepted wisdom attributed all strength and nourishment to meat, he advocated raw fruit and vegetables.

Up to then, little was known of him. His manner was stiff, and his pince-nez and well-trimmed beard were conventional enough to inspire confidence. The few colleagues who had chanced to get to know him and talk to him smiled indulgently at his ideas on nutrition, on raw foods, on 'life force', on 'the roots of disease'. 'He's young,' they said. 'When he gets to our age, when he's had some experience, he'll get over it. We've seen lots like him.' They knew he had converted a modest chalet outside the city into a kind of small clinic, where he could lodge and treat a few patients, but this they considered an indication of commercial rather than medical ambition – a reassuring sign, in fact. But now, this perfectly ordinary man, wearing the same kind of dark suit as themselves, had suddenly emerged as a revolutionary, a medical heretic, a subversive. Not only did he have crazy views about food, but he was actually claiming that the causes of illness lay as much in the patient's mind or soul as in his body, if not more so. He believed that before diagnosing the disease the patient's state of mind must be taken into account and the two things dealt with together. The whole doctor–patient relationship must be re-examined.

Today there is a name for this: psychosomatic medicine. But in 1900 the word 'psychosomatic' did not exist and the link between mind and body in illness was only dimly realised. Bircher-Benner had arrived at this point by his own peculiar route, which was both empirical and experimental. Various incidents in his own life had set him wondering, had triggered off his questing and inventive mind. The circumstances of his own birth were the cause of one of his first and most important discoveries, since they directed his research towards what he came to call the 'life force'.

Max Bircher was born in 1867 in the little Swiss town of Aarau. He was two months premature and was so frail that he was not expected to live. According to the family doctor, the weakness of the child's heart made the future highly problematical – even if he survived, he would probably be a permanent invalid.

But survive he did. He grew into a quiet, thoughtful, well-behaved child. When his mother saw him hand in hand with his brother, ten months older and bursting with health, she felt anxious for the spindly little fellow, frowning, struggling, panting, in his efforts to keep up, but never letting go. 'What willpower!' she thought. But as well as willpower, he felt something else bubbling up inside him – that 'life force', the source of vitality and good health, that was to become the linchpin of his thinking, the springboard for his experiments and discoveries.

Long before the age of reason, Max knew he was different. His brother could run fast, jump high, climb trees, and lift with ease weights that seemed enormous to him. He was always being told, 'No, Max, that's too hard for you. . . . You're not strong enough, you can't go with him. . . . It's time for your rest. . . . Be careful.'

But his whole being rejected this inferiority. Looking in the mirror, it seemed that, apart from being pale and thin, there was no basic difference between him and his brother: he had two legs and two arms attached to the same sort of body. Logically, then, they should be able to do the same things. When no one was looking, he would grip hold of a boulder his brother had been playing with, tensing his hands, getting red in the face, digging his feet into the grass – but the stone didn't budge. He would run till he was out of breath, till his heart was hammering, and he was almost collapsing – and find he had only gone a few yards. So he sat down to ponder upon the strength that eluded him.

Ten years later, his mother marvelled to see him, a captain of artillery in the military cadets, leading marches and manoeuvres, coming home on a Sunday after a day's hill-walking and rock-climbing, or getting in late after a long evening spent playing the drums in an orchestra. He gave piano lessons to a few pupils, too, while studying at the Aarau high school, and still found time to be president of the students' association, and to learn Russian. To his family, it seemed like a miracle.

To Max it was a victory – his first victory over illness, for a body that cannot do what one wants it to do is an ill body. But how did he achieve it? At an age when most of us are guided only by instinct, he was thinking things out. With tenacity and courage, he used every discipline available to him – gymnastics, walking, mountain-climbing in all weathers, plunging into freezing water and swimming. Intuitively, he used the forces of nature – air, sun and water. He willed and worked himself into health, driving himself harder than he was ever to allow any patient of his to do.

He never really decided to become a doctor; he just knew that that was what he would do. His mother believed that the origin of this vocation dated back to when he was only two years old. She had had a fall, and her leg was badly cut and bleeding profusely. Max had not seemed frightened or upset, but had watched every movement of the doctor's as he stitched up the wound. Though she had herself been too frightened to watch, she gained a strange sense of confidence from his calm and interested gaze. She was reminded of this incident some time later, when she found him cutting out little paper figures and removing their arms and legs, which he then carefully stuck on again with glue. So well did he mimic the movements and manner of the doctor that he was nicknamed the Little Doctor, and his family felt sure that it was not just play-acting, that he was really trying to understand how people could be cured. Though frail children generally tend to be more thoughtful and observant than their more energetic fellows, his mother's accident does seem to have had a great effect on Max.

As he grew into adolescence, he worked hard to become a doctor; everything he thought or did was directed to that aim. Life itself gave him a training. It took no devious searching to find the way; all he had to do was to open his eyes, and he was very good at doing that. (Doctor Bircher-Benner's look was to be famous – an ice-blue gaze that gave the impression of seeing bodies and minds with

X-ray vision and, even from behind his pince-nez, conveyed fatherly tenderness and compassion.)

But at the end of the summer of 1885 Max's dreams crashed about his ears. His father died, leaving a widow and five children, but no money. His sisters were young, and his elder brother, not much older than he was, could not shoulder the entire responsibility. How could he possibly carry on with his studies?

He became so worried that he could not sleep. This effect of the mind on the body was to influence his thinking considerably later on – the fact that his worry was making him an insomniac, and thus a sick man. For the moment, however, his insomnia set him off along a different route. Accept it he would not. Sure at first that it was only temporary, he tried to tire himself out every evening with work or reading, but to no avail. He was still tossing and turning all night. He was determined to overcome this in the same way as he had earlier forced himself into good health, but all his efforts of will had the opposite effect; his nervous tension kept him awake till dawn, and he learnt to his cost that willpower is not everything. So he finally gave in, and went to see his family doctor.

The doctor assured him that it was not serious and prescribed sleeping tablets. When they did not work he prescribed a stronger drug – enough, he assured Max, to put an ox to sleep. An ox maybe, but not Max. The doctor tried every known hypnotic, without success. In despair, he finally suggested trying something more unusual: he told Max to go out that evening to a bar, and drink eight glasses of beer in rapid succession. This Max did, though he didn't enjoy it much, but that night was the worst ever: he didn't have even the brief sleep in the early hours that had kept him going up to then. He had now tried everything, and could only resign himself to managing as best he could on the minimal amount of sleep he could get.

One morning, however, he performed so badly at his riding lesson that the instructor was appalled: 'What's the matter with you, Bircher? You look terrible, your legs are wobbling, your hand is shaking. Have you been out on the tiles all night?'

When Max explained that for weeks he had hardly slept, the instructor made a surprising suggestion: 'Try Priessnitz's wet packs – they work on me.'

Max had never heard of Priessnitz, and the treatment sounded extremely odd, but at least it was natural. That night he took a sheet down to the courtyard, soaked it in the freezing water of the outside cistern, wrung it out and went to his bedroom. He spread the wet sheet on top of his bed-covers, lay down on it and carefully rolled himself up in it. Its cold wetness was a shock, but within minutes it turned into a delightful relaxing warmth, and in a quarter of an hour he was sleeping peacefully. Hydrotherapy, which was to be of such importance in his medical practice, had come into his life.

But his worries had not eased. His family could not possibly pay for his medical studies. He was determined not to give up, however, and in the end various friends came to his mother's assistance, and his godfather was able to lend Max just enough money to see him through his studies at Zurich University Medical School.

He was excited by his first introduction to biology and physiology, and resolved to learn all there was to know about the discoveries of the period. He felt sure that the key to the secret of life was to be found in science. His clinical studies, on the other hand, were a disappointment. But when he complained to his fellow students, he was amazed to find that they didn't agree.

'But can't you see how superficial all our medical work is?' he said. 'We spend nine-tenths of our time learning pathological description, and just rush through the diagnostics. We're only interested in appearances – I'm quite sure the secondary symptoms are often the important ones. They can point to a complication that's far more serious than the illness we're actually treating.'

'What do you mean, Max? You can't treat what you can't see!'

'No, no. It's the submerged part of the iceberg that matters. That's where the real causes of the illness are.'

They teased him: 'All right, then, you dive in! And if you get to the bottom and back, you can tell us what you find. We're here to cure the visible, not the invisible.'

'It'll be a miracle if you ever cure anything at all, with your hit-and-miss prescriptions.'

'We save a lot more people here at the hospital than we lose. That's what counts.'

'And what happens to all those people when they get home? Do we know whether they get ill again, and if so, why? We should follow them up. What happens when a patient has left us is what we should be interested in. That really shows what we've done for them.'

'Well, if that's your idea of medicine, you'll never get rich. Following patients home – you're mad! You couldn't do it in a lifetime!'

Such arguments left him unmoved. He had his own ideas about illness, and the role of medicine. In fact, what concerned him most was not so much aftercare as what happened before. He wanted to know the *causes* of illness. Why do people get ill? Is a patient's past a help or a hindrance to recovery? How can an organism be regenerated? These were the questions he wanted to answer.

Bircher's ideas made little impression on his professors or his fellow students, who all stuck to their hallowed traditions. His questions did not interest them. Students were there to learn how to tell one illness from another, and to accept that when an illness has been diagnosed and the correct prescription given (which usually cures it), the doctor's job is over.

He never really fitted into the medical pattern either. He had never enjoyed the heavy drinking most of the students indulged in and, under the influence of Professor Auguste Forel,[1] he determined to give up alcohol altogether. This set him apart – his fellow students took to ignoring him, and even the waitresses in the refectory would laugh at him and refuse to give him water. This experience taught him an invaluable lesson: to value his own opinion more than other people's. The absurdity of the situation helped him make it a rule to abide by his own discoveries and convictions, even when they were in conflict with accepted views.

In 1891 he completed his course, and received his diploma as a doctor of medicine in Zurich. He was twenty-four. The more he thought about it, the more convinced he became that a doctor does not only need knowledge; he must have intuition, a sixth sense to penetrate beyond clinical appearances that may conceal the real root of the trouble, to see beyond what he can know. He felt at once ignorant and self-assured. He knew that he was going to seek for truth, and that truth lay in Nature – the nature both of man and of his environment, the two being complementary. But he had no idea where that search would lead him.

Time was passing. He must repay his debts, which meant starting to practise, and he was anxious to begin. But, painfully aware how much he still had to learn, he gave himself a few months' grace, which he spent with the famous physiologist, Max Rubner, in Berlin. When he

---

[1]Auguste Forel (1848–1931), a Swiss doctor and internationally known psychiatrist, became Director of the Zurich Mental Asylum. He produced an outstanding work on the subject of ants, *Le monde social des fourmis du globe comparé à celui des hommes.*

returned to Zurich he realised that, even had he been able to afford it, he had no inclination to set up in a fashionable district where he would be treating the ailments of the overfed and the capricious nerves of rich women. He established his consulting-room in a densely populated suburb where most of his patients were Swiss or Italian immigrant workers in the local factories. They never came to the doctor until the last possible moment, and Bircher was continually made aware of the ravages caused by poor nutrition: they had too little food, and their diet was anything but balanced, yet they had to meet the physical demands of hard manual work. His patients were seldom ill from overeating, only the reverse. Malnutrition robbed their bodies of all their natural defences.

One evening he opened his door to a woman in a shawl and apron. A small child, its eyes too large, its skin transparent, was clinging to her skirts. The woman's pale face and discoloured eyelids told him everything, but he listened as she described her sense of total exhaustion. She had five children. Her husband worked at nights, and she worked during the day. There was no need to examine her. Bircher took a gold coin from his purse and gave it to her: 'This is what you need – all of you – to eat a proper meal. You don't need medicine, just good meat.' After she had gone, he thought deeply. Meat is expensive, beyond the means of most people. Is meat the *only* source of strength and energy, the *only* source of good health?

The wretchedness he saw day after day was not purely physiological, though it always became so. An instance was the alcoholic who threatened him with an axe. The man's wife had left him, and he had started drinking to forget. The drink had turned him into a sick man, but it was only his despair that had made him take to drink in the first place. Bircher was left with the idea (which later became a certainty) that it is the sick mind or soul that drags the body along with it. It is seldom the body that gets ill first. Were it not for the errors of their parents, most children would be born healthy; the chains of heredity are a weight drawing people down towards disease. He was not absolutely sure of these things, but they were theories he found attractive, and more and more compelling. He was to be in practice for four years and be ill himself before the ideas he had been groping for about the vital power of food took definite shape. It was only then he began to use raw foods as part of his treatment.

Even in his early years, he became so well known among the poor that there were often long queues at his door. But despite all his visits and consultations, and his own research, he still found the time to meet and fall in love with a young woman from Alsace, Elisabeth Benner, daughter of a pharmacist from Mulhouse. They married in 1893, and he followed the Swiss-German tradition of adding her surname to his: he was now Max Bircher-Benner. Elisabeth was lively, intelligent and spirited. In ten years she bore seven children, four boys and three girls.

They had been happily married for two years when Max had jaundice very badly. He lay in bed, miserable and so nauseated by the milky diet prescribed that he refused to eat at all. Elisabeth was very frightened – no one could go on without food day after day. One afternoon she was peeling apples to stew when she suddenly looked at a sliver of the fruit in her hand and wondered if he could eat that. He liked it, and it didn't make him sick. Over the next few days she got him to eat several apples in tiny pieces. Once he was better, however, he did not give it another thought – it was just one of those odd fancies the sick sometimes have. If it had been one of his patients, he would probably have been more observant.

Just a month later, he became very concerned over a girl patient of his, and happened to meet a doctor friend to whom he talked about the case. The girl had, he said, become progressively incapable of digesting any food, however light or bland. 'Food that has been completely ground up and strained, that she has swallowed as a soup at night, remains in precisely the same state when we draw it out of her stomach in the morning – no digestion at all has taken place, there is no trace of gastric juice. She is going to starve to death. I've tried everything.'

His colleague thought for a moment, and then replied, 'How can one ever be sure one has tried *everything*? I once found in a textbook an extraordinary prescription of Pythagoras for digestive troubles: a purée of raw fruit, mixed with a little honey and goat's milk. According to the author, it worked wonders. Why not try that on your patient?'

'Raw fruit – in a stomach that isn't functioning at all?'

'Well, it can't make things any worse than they are, can it?'

Bircher-Benner spent half the night thinking about this curious suggestion. To give raw food would go against everything he had been taught. Surely anything uncooked would be even heavier, even harder to digest? And Pythagoras was hardly a recognised authority. Then he suddenly remembered the apple he had eaten himself.

The next morning he suggested it to his patient, and she agreed to try. The mixture was pleasant-tasting and refreshing – the first thing she had enjoyed for a long time. Her stomach did not reject it, and the following day his examination showed that she had digested it – the first food she had digested for several weeks. (Enzymes had not yet been discovered, and it was not realised that the action of various enzymes enables raw fruit to digest itself, as it were, without help from the gastric juices.) Bircher-Benner gradually increased the quantity of fruit, and cautiously introduced vegetables as well, until finally the girl's digestive system was functioning normally again. After this, he was able to add other foods to her diet. In later life she always spoke of him as her saviour, and it is interesting to note that she lived to the age of seventy-five with no further digestive problems.

Bircher-Benner had still to decide whether her cure was pure chance, or whether he had made a scientific discovery. Comparing it with his own experience of the apples, he found the two cases similar and the results identical. Could there be some curative quality in raw fruit and vegetables that was destroyed by cooking? If so, what was it? The suggestion was in complete contradiction to all accepted ideas: the chemical changes caused by cooking were supposed to make food *more* digestible, not less. Was he mad? Was it possible that doctors and scientists could have been wrong for so long? Could a young doctor of twenty-eight really have made such a discovery? Other people must surely have had such ideas, but he didn't know how to begin finding out who they might be. After some thought, he realised that two cases, however overwhelming, were not enough. He must write out an account of what had happened, and then compare it with further observations, working out cause and effect by scientific method.

He used his own family as guinea-pigs – first himself, then his wife, then the children. When the results were undeniable, he approached his patients and asked them to collaborate in what he admitted was a series of tests and experiments. His dossier grew. It was clear that he had made a discovery: raw fruit and vegetables did have unique curative powers. When traditional remedies failed, diseases of the digestive system could be treated and cured by raw food – which Bircher-Benner was soon to describe as 'living' food.

It was a revolution, but not one he could carry through

alone. He needed to find backing for his statements, to find other people working on the same lines. Perhaps there were people who had got further than he had. He spent his evenings and part of each night studying. He consulted books on nutrition, chemistry and physics; he ransacked the library in vain. He must find a theoretical basis for what his experiments had shown him; empiricism in medicine will not do.

Finally his mind was made up. He closed his consulting-room, moved his wife and children to Mulhouse to be near her parents and, in 1897, set off for Vienna. He wanted to meet Sigmund Freud, who was giving lectures in the medical faculty there. Freud's studies might seem very different from his own, but to Bircher-Benner, medicine was a whole. Raw fruit, though it worked wonders, could not be a panacea for all ills, but only part of that whole. Every sick person was a complex being who must have a complete treatment if the illness was to be cured. Freud's work showed Bircher-Benner a new approach to illness: not just the illnesses of the mind, the brain, the nerves – what we today call mental illness – but all illness, because the psychological element is always vital. Though it seems obvious today, in those days such a notion was generally dismissed as diabolically-inspired heresy.

After attending Freud's lectures on psychotherapy, Bircher-Benner had a number of private conversations with him, and these provided him with a framework for his psychological understanding of the sick. From Professor Winternitz he learnt the beginnings of hydrotherapy. From Lahmann in Dresden and Rubner in Berlin – both outstanding physiologists and dieticians – he was able to widen the knowledge he had managed to amass so far. He was now ready to return to Zurich, where he opened a small sanatorium in a six-bedroom chalet on the slopes of Zurichberg, not as a money-making venture but to enable him to carry on his research; with his patients on the spot, he could pursue each case to its conclusion.

In 1899 he discovered the principle that explained the curative power of raw fruit and vegetables, which he christened 'living matter'. This was the second law of thermodynamics (following Carnot and Clausius), recognised today by the Nobel-prize-winning physicist Erwin Schrödinger as the law that governs nutrition. It was this discovery that caused him to be excommunicated from the scientific establishment of his own time and country, and that excommunication marked the beginning of the new life of Max Bircher-Benner.

# 3. Success

The word 'clinic' is perhaps too grand a name for the small house where my father lived with his family in 1900. He took in only a few patients, and on them he was able to try out his nutritional principles and continue his research. The house was given the appropriate name of 'Force de Vie', Life Force. The doctors in Zurich, when questioned about it, would reply with heavy sarcasm that it was just a family boarding-house where they were stingy with the food. They would point out, even more unpleasantly, that 'Bircher' (now never called Doctor) could not afford to make any mistakes: he would be wise to avoid taking on anyone seriously ill, because at the slightest hint of any negligence there would be trouble.

It must be remembered that at this time Bircher-Benner had very few friends, especially among his colleagues. Most of his friends were his patients, and indeed it was his patients' needs that led him to set up the clinic. Instead of prescriptions and complicated medication, he offered them rules for healthy living and a revolutionary system of diet. It is much easier to get patients to swallow drugs than to change bad habits which they may well have had since childhood, but it was only by following his dietary rules strictly that they could be helped. The same applies today. It is only too easy to fall into bad eating habits at home, simply because they *are* easy. Bircher-Benner found that his patients had to be in the right frame of mind to respond to his treatment, and so he supervised them closely, varying the treatment according to their reaction. His medicine was experimental, and observation was a vital part of it.

For this reason, and also for reasons of economy, he decided to live with his family in the lower part of the house, leaving the three upper floors for the patients. It was a far cry from the commercial enterprise which some of his colleagues accused him of operating. Bircher-Benner ran the house himself, with the help of his wife and his sister, and fees for the small number of patients were moderate. His ambition, as we have seen, was not to make money but to establish a centre for a way of life which he hoped would be widely accepted. Though he might have only six patients now, tomorrow he would have a hundred. He thought big, and he thought ahead.

It was not an age of publicity, of course, and in any case he could not have afforded to advertise – yet within six months there were more applicants than his clinic could hold. They were all people whose cases had been given up as hopeless by practitioners of traditional medicine, so they had nothing to lose, and hoped perhaps to gain some slight strength for living. The word passed round that there was a peculiar sanatorium just outside Zurich where illness was treated by natural means. From all sides, amazed witnesses reported on this 'extraordinary nursing home' with its eccentric treatment.

In November 1906, Mademoiselle Cécile D. stood gazing with distaste around her clinic bedroom with its spartan, functional furniture. She had been caring for her anaemia and delicate health in various sanatoriums and nursing homes in sunny southern climes. The last doctor she had seen had warned her that it would be a long time before she would be strong enough to return to the harsh winds and the fogs of Switzerland – yet here she was, at the insistence of an uncle who had overridden the protestations of her parents. He told them of the miracles effected by a diet of raw food in Doctor Bircher-Benner's sanatorium, and when her father objected that Cécile loathed raw food, and would simply lose weight from not eating, her uncle replied that a few pounds' weight lost would be nothing if she could regain her strength. So her father took her there. Dr Bircher-Benner gave the girl a long and detailed examination, and then warned her father that they could not hope for a rapid cure. This is her own account:

I felt depressed and discouraged when my father left. He would come back for me in a few weeks or months, and everything would go on as before. The rules of the place seemed to me to be the last straw: get up at six, wash, and go for a walk. 'But I can't. The doctors say I must spend the morning in bed!'

'Not here, Mademoiselle. But you can go back to bed after breakfast.'

I *knew* I couldn't do it, and I thought, 'I'll collapse, and then they'll realise I was right.' My arms and legs felt like jelly when I got up – I could hardly walk round my bedroom, let alone go into the woods. But when I had taken a few steps outside I breathed deeply and the fresh air smelt good. There was a fine view of Zurich waking up, and to my surprise I walked slowly for twenty minutes. Breakfast was less of a success: I was given a kind of porridge, 'muesli', and the very look of it made me feel sick. Just this once, they said, I could have a cup of milk instead.

It was strange, and my own reactions were contradictory. After breakfast I had a bath, then finally went back to bed. I let them take me to the laboratory, then I had an hour's gymnastics. Everything seemed like a dream. I found the food uneatable and barely touched it. With so much exercise and so little food, I was sure it was only a matter of time till I broke down completely. One morning after a terrible night I was sure that time had come. I buried myself under my eiderdown and, when the nurse came in to ask why I was not outside walking, I said, 'I

'I can't. I've got terrible cramp in my legs.' She nodded
and disappeared. 'At last,' I thought, 'they realise that I'm
not like their other patients.'

Then the door opened, and there was Dr Bircher-
Benner. He came over to my bed, and stroked his beard
thoughtfully. I suddenly felt a wave of confidence.
Everything was going to be different now. His eyes
sparkled with curiosity:

'What's the matter? A broken leg? A hernia? Get up,
and let's see if you can stand.'

I got up and he took my arm. 'Can you walk?' We
walked slowly round the room. 'A walk in the fresh air
would be better,' he said.

'I can't. I'm really ill. I couldn't stand it.'

'I know how lovely it is to be lazy and stay in bed – but
the best thing for cramp is exercise.' He looked me
straight in the eye: 'It's lucky that you don't come from a
working-class family, where a girl of your age can't please
herself. She has to earn her living, ill or not. I've thought
of just the thing to make you forget how rotten you feel –
a lot better than staying in bed.' The tone of his voice
became one of command. 'I'll expect you in the kitchen in
an hour's time. There are a lot of vegetables to prepare.'

'What kind of a doctor is he?' I thought angrily. 'Not a
word of sympathy, no examination. I'll never give him
another chance to ridicule me like that. And if I collapse
he'll have to answer for it!'

But I went to the kitchen and peeled the vegetables and
survived the shock quite well. At my next consultation, Dr
Bircher-Benner asked me anxiously how I felt. 'Better, I
hope?'

'No worse.'

'Exactly. And how do you like our hydrotherapy?'

'The hot baths are nice, but the cold showers are
terrible. I really can't stand it – I can't breathe!'

'You poor girl, that shows how much you need them. You'll have to put up with them for a long time before you're well enough to enjoy them. Anyway, I hope that at least you're eating something?'

I sensed another trap, but I didn't care. 'I don't enjoy it – it's all so tasteless.'

'Still, it nourishes you.'

'Well, I need it to keep me going, with all these exercises.'

He nodded sympathetically: 'I do understand. It's going to take a long time to learn to enjoy the food, too. But *I* am in no hurry, even if you are. All I want is for you to be capable of coping with life when you leave here – mentally *and* physically. However long it takes.'

In the end, it wasn't as long as I had expected. But it was only afterwards that I really saw what Dr Bircher-Benner had taught me. He had strengthened my will to live and developed my energy by showing me that I could work in spite of being so weak. And his regime really regenerated my body.

I am now ninety-two, and as I look back on my life I realise how rich it has been. My four children are all married, and I have seventeen grandchildren. And for all this I have Dr Bircher-Benner to thank; he made me what I am because he didn't just give me a temporary cure, but attacked the roots of my illness.

Madame B. came to visit us at the clinic at the age of eighty, and told us how she, too, owed her health to Dr Bircher-Benner. Sixty years earlier, the medical profession had given her up and she had come to his first clinic. 'He supervised us with the persistence and obstinacy that mark the great doctor. Really, I suppose, it was because he didn't trust us. If a patient didn't follow his orders to the letter, he wouldn't hesitate to tell him to leave, so that his room could go to someone who really wanted to get better.'

Madame B. suffered from an almost total paralysis of the bowels. Doctors had prescribed stronger and stronger laxatives, and they were having less and less effect. Her stay in Zurich began with an unpleasant shock. Dr Bircher-Benner took away all her medicines, and totally changed her diet, making her eat things she had always been forbidden. But she trusted him: he was so careful and so scrupulous, and she knew that if he made a mistake he would have admitted it honestly. So, bravely, she went ahead. After three and a half months in the clinic, she was completely cured. Everyone thought it was a miracle, except Bircher-Benner himself. As he told Madame B., the reason he had such confidence in his treatments was that he had tried them all on himself.

Another anecdote will illustrate his response to emergencies. One day I received a telephone call telling me that a friend was extremely ill.

'What's the matter?' asked my father, when he saw my shocked look.

'My friend Anne is dying. She's almost unconscious and her body is going blue. They are giving her sedatives. She's completely shattered because her engagement has been broken off.'

'Nonsense,' he said. 'No unhappy love affair ever made a woman as ill as that. I'll go and see her.' When we got there, he immediately diagnosed an embolism. Rather than wasting time by calling an ambulance, he gently and carefully lifted Anne into his own car. I drove. When he examined her at the clinic, his diagnosis was confirmed. The treatment was quite simple:

1 Complete bed rest, to prevent the clot moving to the heart.

2 No meat, because animal fats cause the blood to coagulate.

3 Alternating hot and cold sponging, to increase the elasticity of the veins and so improve circulation.

4 A fresh, invigorating diet.

In three weeks, Anne was up and about; the danger was over.

Bircher-Benner's successes became so well known that 'hopeless' cases came to the Zurich clinic as one might go to Lourdes. One day he had a visit from a man whose leg was already black and becoming gangrenous. He had been ordered to have it amputated, but the thought terrified him. My father assured him that he would be able to keep it. He treated him as follows:

1 No alcohol, as it hardens the vein tissue.

2 No meat. Fresh food (fruit and vegetables) only.

3 Gymnastic exercise to stimulate the circulation.

4 Hydrotherapy: alternating hot and cold showers to restore the elasticity of the veins.

The treatment took a year. The cure was considered miraculous. When the man was complimented on his patience, all he said was, 'What's a year, compared with a lifetime?'

In 1911, the by now considerably enlarged clinic employed five doctors, one of whom was a psychotherapist, and a dozen nurses. Seventy patients from all parts of the globe were housed in the main building and its annexes, all prepared to submit to the vigorous discipline of the treatment. It was Bircher-Benner's conviction that to accept illness as though it were fate was to prepare a fertile soil for it. Far from agreeing with the common notion that healthy people are only those who do not *know* what is wrong with them, he insisted that health was the natural state of human beings, and his patients had to work towards that state.

Even people who were used to commanding, rather than obeying, were prepared to undergo his treatments. The fame of his clinic reached the court of the Tsar. One morning several members of the Romanov family made a noisy entrance into the main building. Their complaint was toxic goitre. They were accustomed to eating a lot, drinking a lot and smoking a lot, and they protested loudly when Bircher-Benner, having examined them, prescribed a draconian regime. They were nobles – why should they be treated like moujiks? They weren't being treated like nobles or moujiks, replied the doctor, merely like patients.

They appeared to submit. They got up at six, took long walks in the woods, disported their masses of fat and muscle under the shower, and chewed their raw vegetables with gusto. However, when Bircher-Benner was passing their window a few days later he caught a whiff of Havana tobacco. He looked in and saw the gentlemen drinking and eating merrily. They had sent their servants to buy provisions in Zurich. Enraged, he went into the house and pushed open the door of their room. They looked up in surprise. One, slightly tight, had the supreme effrontery to offer him a glass of vodka. Bircher-Benner, like a bearded prophet of old, pointed to the door:

'You belong in the hotel, not here. I have patients waiting for your rooms. You can go!' And they went. (Detractors who claimed that Bircher-Benner was out for money would have been surprised.)

Three days later, however, their repentant excellencies were back, beating their breasts. Heaven is supposed to rejoice more over the repentant sinner than the just: Bircher-Benner's eye twinkled with sardonic joy behind his glasses, but his face remained severe, and he allowed them back only after they had sworn to behave properly. In fact, the Russian aristocracy eventually became some of the clinic's most ardent propagandists.

The treatment was certainly rigorous, but there were amusements too. Thomas Mann, author of *The Magic Mountain*, captured the spirit of the clinic very well in a letter he wrote to a friend while actually staying there:

> I received your letter under the oddest circumstances in Zurich, in the sanatorium of Dr Bircher-Benner, where one is made to get up at six and lights must be out by nine. It's hard going. At first I kept looking at my suitcases, wrestling with the temptation to leave. However, though Voltaire is more in my line than Rousseau, I'm not sorry I stuck it out. My hitherto intractable digestion has improved in the most extraordinary way, as never before. And my stay here has been enjoyable both for the pleasant company, and the beautiful situation. I shall never forget some of the lighting effects at night. . . .

Bircher-Benner was severe when it came to anything that might interfere with the effectiveness of his treatment or be a hazard to health. But he believed that the more people's minds could be opened to the world, the more harmoniously would their bodies develop. He was a fine musician, and with us, his children, he formed a small chamber orchestra. Max, the eldest, was a pianist, Franklin a cellist, Willy and I played the violin and Ralph the flute. Sometimes we played in the evenings to entertain the patients before they went to bed. There was dancing too, on occasions. My father was a good dancer, and if he saw a woman sitting by herself, he would ask her to dance with him. If she replied that she couldn't dance, he would berate her:

'No wonder you find life depressing if you don't take advantage of its pleasures. The foundations of good health are happiness and a sense of well-being. How can you create a good life for yourself or anyone else if you're going to be a melancholy, embittered, solitary hypochondriac?'

One woman to whom he spoke in this vein suggested that he should write on all his treatment-sheets, 'Dancing classes obligatory.' 'I'll consider it,' he replied.

He certainly had the *joie de vivre* that he recommended to others. At sixty-five he decided to learn modern dance steps, and when jazz first made its timid appearance in Switzerland he was delighted by it and played the drums in jazz concerts.

The 1914–18 war was a difficult period for the clinic, of course, and about a third of its activities had to be cut out. But its international reputation was now assured. Its success was complete. A large building had been put up to house the most modern installations, including a radiography room and hydrotherapy equipment. There was a drawing-room, a dining-room and a concert hall.

Bircher-Benner was incessantly reviewing what he knew and revising his conclusions. When the medical world was beginning to take up the theories of Sigmund Freud, he had already left them behind: he saw psychoanalysis as no more than a small facet of the jewel of truth. It would be as misguided to build an entire system upon it as to ignore it. He saw that a great deal of it led to a dead end, so he could not make it the backbone of his theory of treatment as he had hoped. It could be no more than a reinforcement in his attack on the hidden root of illness – in the soul. He used the word 'soul' in a broad sense, closer to philosophy than religion, though the religious dimension was not excluded. It was undoubtedly his parallel research into the soul that led him to correspond with Mahatma Gandhi, and to produce a major work on the human psyche which appeared in two volumes in 1925 and 1926.[1]

[1]*Der Menschenseele Not.* The sixth edition was published in Zurich in 1953 (*Wendepunktbücher*, no. 8).

Though the Force de Vie clinic acquired such a special reputation among the sick, traditional medical circles took a very different view. But, typically, Bircher-Benner behaved with great honour towards his colleagues. Despite urging from all sides, he refused to write articles or give lectures for the general public about his theories and experiments. He felt that would be unprofessional, and was sure his fellow doctors would ultimately have to recognise the value of his ideas and methods. In this he was perhaps naïve, but not naïve enough to sit back and wait for them to do so. He wanted to instruct his patients and students in the prevention of illness. So he decided to establish a monthly review, *Der Wendepunkt im Leben und im Leiden,* 'The Turning-point in Life and Suffering'. 'The review has now been in existence for over fifty years, and it is still edited by his son Ralph, who used to work with him.' Its earliest readers were mainly his patients. Those who wanted to gain a deeper understanding of Bircher-Benner's principles subscribed to it, and on returning home would lend it to friends in the hope of making more converts. They would also ask their own doctors troublesome questions, which meant that the doctors too had to find out more about Bircher-Benner's ideas, if only to refute them. Not all doctors wore blinkers, and gradually more and more of them subscribed to the *Wendepunkt,* while some even wrote for it. The barrier of hostility was broken down at last.

Medical journals asked Bircher-Benner to contribute articles, and he was invited to put forward his theories at congresses. Though not everyone was instantly converted, attitudes had changed, and the effects were to be considerable. It was not until 1930, thirty years after his excommunication by the medical establishment, that Bircher-Benner's theories began to be internationally accepted, even though they were restoring the health of so many people. Medical authorities, notably in England, France, Germany, Austria, Italy, the USA – and even in Switzerland – began to recommend his work.

One final anecdote illustrates especially well the basis of Bircher-Benner's philosophy and treatment. One day a certain Monsieur J. D. came to him in a state of near collapse. 'What is your job?' asked Bircher-Benner.

'I was an accountant,' replied Monsieur J. D., 'but I can't even work any more. I can't digest anything, so I'm too weak.'

He did indeed look extremely ill – pale, hollow-cheeked, a living skeleton. When he undressed, Bircher-Benner nodded compassionately as he saw the swollen stomach. Examination revealed a serious abdominal ptosis, with all the organs – stomach, liver and spleen – dangerously low. The man was only thirty-seven. 'You realise, doctor, that I've seen a lot of other specialists. I've been told that I need an operation, and that I'll then have to wear a truss for support if I want to go back to work.'

'Well, it's taken you some years to get as bad as this. Would you have the patience to wait a few more months – perhaps even longer – to get better?'

'Without an operation?'

'What I propose is a cure.'

'Must I go into your clinic?'

'No. I haven't got a room for you, and I want you to start treatment at once. You are to follow the diet sheet I give you faithfully. We'll combine that with massage, cold showers, gymnastic exercise and an hour's walk every morning.'

'But I can hardly walk at all,' protested Monsieur J. D. 'I have to lie down after meals or else I'm violently sick.'

'Don't worry,' said Bircher-Benner. 'With my treatment you won't be sick any more. If you find an hour too much, start with half an hour.'

When he saw the prescribed diet, Monsieur J. D.'s face fell. 'But I've been forbidden all raw fruit and vegetables,' he said.

'Well,' said Bircher-Benner firmly, 'I forbid you anything else.'

Three weeks later, the man returned, looking a little better. He said he could walk without too much trouble, and, though his abdomen was still swollen and painful, he was not vomiting. Bircher-Benner extended his diet, adding whole cereals and milk: he also recommended more walks, though warning against over-fatigue.

Monsieur J. D. did not come back. No one knew whether he had finally had an operation, or continued with his treatment, or what had happened. Bircher-Benner forgot him. Then one day, two years later, a brisk, healthy-looking man came into his consulting-room. 'You don't recognise me! I'm J. D. – do you remember what a wreck I was? I've come to let you see what you did for me.' His skin was clear, his cheeks had filled out, he was a good colour, his eyes shone, and his stomach was flat, the muscles young and strong. He owed his health to Dr Bircher-Benner, he said, and his stomach and muscles to walking.

'I followed your advice. I soon found myself enjoying walking, and I've walked all over Switzerland, Italy, Austria and Germany. I've just come back from Sweden. I enjoyed it so much that I began to hum, and then to sing – and I find I have quite a good voice. I've discovered nature, too – the beauty of mountains and valleys and plains, flowers and trees, and birds singing. I think sunrise and sunset are the most beautiful things in the world.'

'You didn't enjoy your job, did you?'

'I don't remember telling you that, but it's quite true. I found accountancy boring and depressing.'

'So your illness enabled you to give it up? But you *said* you were anxious to get back to work!'

'Well, I didn't know how else to earn a living.'

'And you do now?'

'You'd be surprised, doctor. I work on farms, wherever I find myself. I don't need much money, because I eat so simply. And I think I've discovered the most effective medicine of all: I'm a happy man.'

There could hardly be a more perfect example. Raw fruit and vegetables (living foods) cured his intestinal trouble. Walking (physical exercise) repaired his abdominal muscles. Air and sunshine contributed to the development of his wasted body. And giving up the job he disliked (the roots of the illness) restored his mental balance and his enjoyment of life.

# 4. The Bircher-Benner Revolution

The early examples of the Bircher-Benner treatment show that his then revolutionary theories rested upon three key ideas: the roots of illness, life force, and living food.

To Max Bircher-Benner, illness was like the moon, with one side visible and the other hidden; or like an iceberg in which the submerged part is larger and more dangerous than the part one can see. Deeply concealed in that hidden part lay the reasons for illness, and as long as those roots of illness were not removed no cure could be anything but superficial. The question to ask was not 'What illness has this patient got?' but rather 'What is he sick of? Others, society, himself? Illness is not a natural human state. Why, then, has he accepted it? Is he actually enjoying it? Why has he taken refuge in illness? Has he perhaps sought this as a way of resolving his problems – introducing new problems to disguise the old ones?' Thinking along these lines was the beginning of a total reassessment of medicine, of medical intervention, and of doctor–patient relations.

Bircher-Benner's belief that curing the illness as it presented itself did not get rid of the cause was based on the principle that illness is not natural to man, but is the result of human error. It seemed to him, therefore, that one must discover the mistakes one has made in life to find the causes of one's illness – a simple-sounding theory that is anything but simple to put into practice.

Very often, however, these mistakes could be traced to one source – food.[1]

[1] I need hardly point out that Dr Bircher-Benner did not blame bad eating habits for idiopathic illnesses, infections, epidemics, diseases caused by bacilli, or hereditary illness.

## THE ROOTS OF ILLNESS

Alice S., aged twenty, was more than 40 lb overweight when she came to see Dr Bircher-Benner. He found that her case was quite a simple one – she ate too much, and what she ate was largely sugar, fat and starch. The strange thing was that she had put on all this extra weight in only a year. Two years earlier, she told him, she had been slim. And, to prove her point, she showed him snapshots of herself radiant in a summer dress in a family group, and arm in arm with a young man.

'You're engaged?' he asked.

'I was.'

'Has the engagement been broken for long?'

'Just over a year. Oh, doctor, he married my best friend!' So this was the root of the problem. Alice S. was compensating for her disappointment by eating. Her family unfortunately had misconceptions about diet, and bad habits to go with them. Her mother kept telling her that one must eat to grow strong. In her household one had to feed a cold, feed a fever, feed a broken heart. Outside food there was no salvation – it was the answer to all life's problems. Nor could Alice herself see much point in getting thin – her life, she felt, was over.

Bircher-Benner knew that it would be easy enough to get Alice's weight down, but that once she was out of the sanatorium and back at home she would put it all back on again, unless she also recovered her mental equilibrium. By the time she was thirty she would be an obese woman who had given up all hope of ever marrying or having a family, and would fall an easy prey to all sorts of destructive psychoses. This must be prevented.

To Bircher-Benner, what was essential if there was to be a genuine cure was to get the machinery of health working again, to stimulate the mechanisms of self-defence and self-healing, to remove the poison from the depths of the system. He called this process an 'order treatment'.

The restoration of order is not something that can be effected overnight with the help of drugs. The longer the disorder has been going on, the longer the cure will take. Body and mind have formed habits which, though damaging, have become comfortable and even pleasant. Successive distortions have produced new interactions, some of which have taken years to establish. To undo these effects takes time. Treatment by natural means, without the short cut of any chemotherapy, can take a very long time, but it does produce spectacular and permanent cures.

## LIFE FORCE

This treatment must not merely cure disease: it must give good health and this means discovering what aspect of the patient's life caused the illness, then mobilizing the patient's own life force to change it. Bircher-Benner's view was that we all have considerable reserves of life force, but they are not inexhaustible. The problem is that we behave as though they were, and squander them. 'Not everyone lives to a ripe old age, but if you do it is surely better to reach it in peak condition.' Having begun his own life handicapped by illness and built up his own health by willpower alone, Bircher-Benner knew better than anyone what we can demand and expect of that force.

He set out to change the face of medicine – which in the 1890s called for a great deal of courage. It was his determination to gain recognition for his theories that made him go on, despite dispiriting times when no one but himself had any faith in them.

When friends referred to the great efforts he had made, he would reply, 'Surely anything is possible if you have life force?' The question was how to conserve this capital, how to restore it once lost, where to get it from. Could everyone hope for this kind of regeneration? In Bircher-Benner's view they could: it is within the reach of all of us. This brings us to the very core of his teaching, one of his most cherished theories: 'A person who eats healthily and whose metabolism[1] is not too high is more susceptible to psychological treatment, because his brain functions better and more clearly. His capacities for coherent thought are greater, and thus he genuinely wants to recover his health. For any change to be permanent, physical and psychological treatments must go hand in hand, the psychological treatment being supported by a healthy diet and a way of life in harmony with the laws of nature.'

## LIVING FOOD

Bircher-Benner's prime precept, from which all the rest followed, can be summed up in the phrase: 'Life comes from life.' Air, sun, water, green vegetables – these are the reservoirs of energy that nature generously places at our disposal. Since a revolution always needs a slogan, his could well be 'Eat living food' – food that is fresh, raw and not processed in any way.

Today, over sixty years later, major research is going on all over the world into the nutritive and curative value of natural food. Yet there are still doctors, trained in traditional academic medicine that has not changed over the last hundred years, who insist that raw food is indigestible, that where there are gastro-intestinal troubles all fruit should be cooked, that the excess of fibre in raw vegetables produces flatulence, and that such food has little nutritive value in any case. None of these statements is true.

---

[1]Metabolism, whose Greek root means 'change', is the series of processes whereby matter is transformed into energy by the body and its cells.

Probably the most spectacular cures produced by this method of dieting are those of ailments of the gastro-intestinal system. Even the most persistent enteritis and the most intractable constipation have been found to yield to a strict diet of raw foods.

As we have seen, it was only gradually, after successive experiments, that Dr Bircher-Benner came to reject traditional ideas. The very fact of asking the question 'What makes raw food more effective? Why does it cure people?' represented the beginnings of the answer. For the essential components of what he called *crudités* (not to be confused with the *crudités* one finds on a restaurant menu) are necessary to life. Vegetables and fruit contain effective antibiotics with no side-effects (one can but regret that the chemical industry has not made more use of nature in this field). They also contain minerals vital to human life, and two elements so important that they alone would justify the Bircher-Benner treatment: enzymes and vitamins.

## ENZYMES

The living cells of vegetables contain many enzymes[1] that produce a kind of self-digestion process, thus making raw vegetables far more digestible than cooked ones. Cabbage is an excellent example: when raw it is highly digestible, with a beneficial effect on gastro-intestinal problems (and also on rheumatism), whereas when cooked it is hard to digest and causes flatulence. This self-digestion due to inherent enzymes represents a considerable saving of energy, and of albumin expenditure. It takes about 8g of enzymes to digest a plate of ordinary food.

But when the enzymes present in raw food are cooked, they disappear completely. Being the kind of proteins they

[1] An enzyme is a substance produced by living cells which promotes chemical change.

are, they are denatured by heat. They work best at a temperature of around 40°C (104°F) and cannot survive anything much above that. A well-balanced diet must therefore include a daily allowance of raw fruit and vegetables, bearing in mind that different varieties have their own different, and often complementary, values.

## VITAMINS

Vegetables and fruit contain most of the vitamins that are essential to life and health, but a healthy diet means getting the proportion right. It is therefore a question of knowing how much of which vitamin each type contains, in order to have the right daily intake (see the Table of Daily Vitamin Requirements, p. 163).

And they must be eaten raw, because cooking destroys a lot of the vitamins. Intense and prolonged heat (such as when a vegetable soup is cooked for over an hour) destroys vitamin A, found in carrots, cabbage, endive, tomatoes. A serious lack of this vitamin is likely to damage the eyesight. Vitamin C – which is in a great many fruits, among them strawberries, raspberries, lemons, oranges, melons, and grapes, and in vegetables such as cabbage, spinach and lettuce – disappears when only slightly heated. Furthermore, most minerals, like iron, magnesium, calcium and potassium, are dissolved in cooking water.

When people suffer serious vitamin deficiency, present-day medicine introduces synthetic vitamins. Interestingly enough, some cannot be synthesised chemically, and have to be extracted from the plants that contain them – for instance, vitamin $D_2$ from ergot of rye. But why should we take in tablet form what we can get so pleasantly from food, and why should we wait for a vitamin deficiency to appear? Surely prevention is better than cure, and vitamins are better found in their natural sources.

Major research is now going on into the changes caused by cooking. W. Ziegelmeyer, a professor and doctor, writes that

> The raw state ensures the preservation of certain nutritive substances, prevents the denaturing of albumin, and maintains mineral substances at their highest concentration. It has been shown that cooking acts on the colloidal state of foodstuffs. It destroys the balance of the large molecules, and changes the nature of the relations among the component parts – the surface tension, the degree of dispersion, the osmotic pressure, the degree of dilution, the differing colloidal states of the molecules, the absorbency or water-resistance of the colloids. It modifies the viscosity and reduces the energy potential. The stronger (i.e. less dispersed) the energies remain in their interactions, the greater will be the total production of energy, and the greater the efficiency. Rubner writes: 'The more intact foods are when entering the body, the more likely they are to fulfil their physiological function.' This is also what Kollath meant when he said: 'Let natural foods stay as natural as possible!'[1]

When Dr Bircher-Benner gave patients their diet-sheets, he never omitted the vital rule that some green vegetables must be eaten daily. He would often add, 'Really green leaves. The white leaves in the heart of the lettuce may be more tender, but they haven't had the sun on them, and I don't think they're worth very much ... In fact, if you're going to throw *any* of it away, that's the part to throw!'

[1] *Unsere Lebensmittel und ihre Veränderungen* (Leipzig, Steinkopf-Verlag).

Hardly any natural food is as rich in vitamins, or has the perfect balance of mineral salts, as green leafy vegetables.[1] Bircher-Benner's advice can be better appreciated when one considers a few examples.

Vitamin A is relatively abundant in all the green parts of a plant – 140g (5 oz) of spinach provides a day's supply of vitamin A (5 mg). It is also to be found in walnuts, whole grain cereal, and natural cold-pressed vegetable oils, especially linseed and sunflower oils.

Green-leaved vegetables contain more vitamin C even than citrus fruits, thought to be the most plentiful source. Cabbage, for example, has twice as much as lemons, and Brussels sprouts two and a half times as much. But this vitamin is extremely sensitive to the effects of air and heat: freshly picked spinach contains more vitamin C than spinach from a shop. Increased amounts of vitamin A (6000–8000 I.U.) plus massive amounts of vitamin C (which must *only* be given under control of a doctor), are very effective in drying out alcoholics and in treating rheumatism, especially rheumatoid arthritis. They are vital in treating the adrenal glands that produce the hormone cortisone, and ACTH. This combination of vitamins also helps resistance to the effects of such stimulants as coffee, makes maximum use of proteins, and helps the nervous system to function effectively. It also intensifies the action of adrenaline, of cathepsin (which organizes the construction of protein), and of vitamin B1 (which calms the nerves).

Vitamin P strengthens the capillaries. It is particularly abundant in spinach and citrus fruits.

[1]Green plant cells contain carotene, which is actually the precursor of vitamin A; in other words, it is transformed into vitamin A in the human body, by the action of unsaturated fatty acids.

Studies at Stanford University have shown that vitamin U[1] plays a vital part in healing gastric and duodenal ulcers. Sufficient quantities of it are found only in green vegetables, and it is extremely sensitive to heat.

Folic acid, a B vitamin (related to vitamin $B_{12}$) which is found mainly in green vegetables, is important for the metabolism and so is vital for good health.

The glycosides in spinach and other vegetables increase the secretion of digestive juices, which is of special importance for children, the sick, pregnant women and convalescents.

There are also the plant oestrogens, which are vital for regulating the reproductive system.

Finally, green vegetables are also rich in mineral salts, whose role is essentially that of rapidly reducing the acid content of the tissues and the saliva. That acidity comes from a diet containing too much starch, flour, fat, protein and sugar. Raw vegetables are thus outstandingly valuable, and the use of raw food as a system of dietary cure is the essence of the Bircher-Benner revolution.

[1]Vitamin U is an unfamiliar specification for DL methylmetheoninsulfonium-chlorid. It is a white, finely grained crystal powder, and very easily water-soluble. It is found in cabbage, lettuce, celery, carrots, tomatoes, yeast. Today it is mostly synthesised. According to Szybo and Vargha (*Arzneimittel-Forschung*, 23 October 1960) Vitamin U is effective against stomach ulcers and is, therefore, called also anti-ulcus vitamin, or ulcus-protective factor.

# 5. Raw Foods, Cereals and Milk Products

To many people, the Bircher-Benner diet system looks like just another vegetarian regime, with nothing new or special about it. But there is a vital difference. A vegetarian could be someone who eats nothing but tinned vegetables and fruit that have lost all the virtues they possessed when alive. And, though animal fats and proteins are excluded from a Bircher-Benner cure, they are not banned altogether once the cure is over, whereas a vegetarian diet would exclude them permanently. (It is nevertheless advisable to eat them only in moderation, and desirable to do without them altogether. However, if giving them up represents too much of a sacrifice, they are permitted, providing they are absolutely fresh and chosen carefully. See Chapter 6.)

## RAW FOODS

Vegetarians make raw vegetables an important part of their diet, but they do not use them in the same way as the Bircher-Benner system does: that is, selectively for a given condition. Every illness treated by those who carry on the Bircher-Benner system (the mainly Swiss or German students of Max Bircher-Benner) is prescribed its own specific diet (see Chapter 10).

But, valuable though a raw food diet is, it cannot provide all the essential nutrients the body needs, and a well-balanced diet must also include cereals and milk products. It must be remembered that a diet of nothing but fruit and vegetables should be followed only under strict medical supervision, and that its function is to be a kind of shock treatment.

A well-balanced meal should be made up of raw fruits and vegetables (about half the meal), followed by cooked foods: wholemeal bread, cereals, potatoes, cooked vegetables, various kinds of soup, soya,[1] sesame seeds, cheese (made from scalded rather than fermented curds), cottage and cream cheeses, fresh butter, vegetable oil, and so on.

## CEREALS

The most important foods after raw fruit and vegetables are cereals, and the most valuable cereal is wheat. But the grain should be eaten whole, including the wheatgerm, which is rich in basic nutrients. Wheatgerm contains 40 per cent albumin (equivalent to 10 per cent of the total protein in wheat);[2] 10–12 per cent fat (equivalent to 20–25 per cent of the total fat in wheat), including the fat-soluble vitamins, especially A and E, and five-sixths of the phospholipid content.[3] Over half the vitamin content is contained in the husks, or bran, of the grain, which are removed during processing. The removal of the wheatgerm during processing means the loss of most of the vitamin B, as well as almost all the delicate taste of the wheat – the nutty taste that develops when it is baked or boiled.

Professor J. C. Drummond, who headed a scientific committee on wartime nutrition in Great Britain, is worth quoting: 'Whole wheat, wheatgerm included, is an

[1] Soya has been known in China for thousands of years. It contains protein and essential fatty acids as well as vitamins B, E and K and a wealth of mineral salts, notably calcium and iron. On the other hand, it contains comparatively little starch, so it is an ideal food for diabetics. It is best used in the form of flour, and to replace eggs.

[2] Mixed with milk and vegetable protein in a proportion of 1 part to 10, wheatgerm albumin provides a perfect balance for our requirement of indispensable albuminoids.

[3] Phospholipids are important for the formation of bones, and for healthy teeth, for the brain and the nerves, as well as for the preservation of the cells' 'filtering action'.

adequate food. And the sooner we manage to get people to eat the whole wheat, the sooner we shall see one of the greatest improvements in human health that mankind has ever witnessed.'

Cereals may be eaten raw or cooked. Here, too, there is a myth to be dispelled. It has long been believed that raw cereals were extremely indigestible, but this is not true, and indeed raw cereals are indispensable to health because of their wealth of nutrients, especially vitamins B and E, and of unsaturated fatty acids. But, though raw cereals are essential, they should be taken only in small quantities: 25–60g (1–2 oz) a day is plenty, preferably eaten in the morning. They need grinding, but a coffee mill or liquidiser can be used for this.

## MILK PRODUCTS

Dairy products have an important place in the Bircher-Benner system but not all are equally important. Non-fermented cooked cheeses are acceptable – Gruyère, Parmesan, Port Salut, and Emmenthal – as well as milk, low-fat soft unfermented cheese (such as cottage cheese, demi-sel, petit-suisse, etc.), buttermilk, yoghourt and sour milk.

After cereals, milk is the most important human food as long as it is not cooked. (100g or 3½ oz of milk contains 3.5g of protein, 3.9g of fat, 4.6g of carbohydrate, as well as vitamins $B_2$, A, D, and C, and calcium.) Heat coagulates the albumin, a moment's boiling destroys the vitamin C, and a temperature of 70°C (175°F) destroys the yeasts that digest fats. This is why raw milk is so much more digestible than boiled. Unfortunately, however, one cannot normally advise people to drink raw milk, even in the country, unless it is known to come from a modern dairy where hygienic conditions are guaranteed: the risks of contamination and tuberculosis are too great. Most of the milk sold is pasteurised and, though this process undoubtedly reduces its quality, it does preserve some of the biological value. But avoid milk that has been sterilised, homogenised or boiled, since all these processes reduce its nutritive value.

The ideal would be for all countries to follow the example of Finland. There, where there is little fruit and fresh vegetables are only available for part of the year, good quality milk is a vital source of nutrients. Over the course of ten years (1925–35), there was a programme of action to ensure that all cattle were healthy, and that dairy installations were so hygienic that raw milk could be drunk without danger.

Fermented milk products like sour milk, low-fat soft cheese and yoghourt, are preferable to boiled milk because lactic bacteria develop faster than others and produce lactic acid, which attacks harmful bacteria. Fermented milk thus avoids the dangers of raw milk without losing its advantages.

## MUESLI

One of the most successful ways of combining cereals, milk products and raw fruit is muesli. As such it is an important part of the Bircher-Benner diet.

Max Bircher-Benner discovered what was to become *Birchermuesli* quite by chance. He was a great walker, attributing his own good health to walking and recommending it as the best and most natural form of exercise. One evening, when walking in the mountains, he happened to arrive at a mountain hut just as the shepherd who lived there was preparing his supper. The shepherd invited him to share his meal – a kind of porridge of coarsely milled wheat in milk, sweetened with honey, which he ate while munching an apple. The doctor had a long talk with him. His father, he said, had got the recipe from *his* father.

'But why the apple?'

He didn't know, but he had noticed that when he went without the apple, the porridge lay heavier on his stomach, and he did not feel so well nourished.

How long had he been eating this food? All his life, he said. And how old was he now? 'Seventy. I've never been to the doctor, and I can climb the hills as well as when I was a young man – I never get out of breath.'

How many times a day did he eat this food? 'Twice a day, morning and evening. At noon I have bread' (a very good wholemeal bread, in fact) 'with apples or perhaps nuts.'

Bircher-Benner's curiosity led him to investigate further, and he discovered that the shepherd's recipe was not original. In the parts of the country where there was plenty of fruit, meals, and especially the evening meal, usually consisted of various cereals – the local German wheat, oats or barley – with raw milk straight from the cow, fruit and sometimes nuts. So he discovered muesli: a mixture of oatmeal and milk, grated apple or fresh berries (strawberries or bilberries). After various experiments, Bircher-Benner introduced it into his diets, and it soon became the staple food of the clinic. Indeed, it acquired a far wider fame: it is served today in England as 'Swiss muesli'; in Milan it has become *Dolce Sorpresa;* and in Zurich one can ask for a Birchermuesli in any hotel or restaurant. Unfortunately, though, the dish you get will, depending on the establishment, be more or less abundantly embellished with thick cream, tinned fruit and sugar, while the apple is left out. In this guise, it preserves none of its original properties. The various types of 'Birchermuesli' you find in packets may have been made with powdered milk, dehydrated apples, raisins, nuts or beet sugar and indeed the only authentic ingredient may be the oatmeal. The best way is to make it up yourself from fresh ingredients.

Muesli is a perfect food, a résumé of the Bircher-Benner diet. The cereals in it (oats, wheat that has been soaked or germinated, millet grains, soya flakes, and so on) contain vitamins A and E, $B_1$, $B_2$, and $B_{12}$, and phosphorus, phospholipids, albumin, and protein. The milk provides vitamin $B_2$, mineral salts, vitamins C and A and fats. The sugar or honey provides iron and carbohydrates. The apples contain potassium, vitamins C and $B_1$, pectin and carbohydrates. The nuts contain protein, potassium, phosphorus, vitamins $B_1$ and $B_2$. Other fresh fruit may also be added. The lemon juice provides vitamin C and potassium.

The Muesli is a special feature of Dr Bircher-Benner's diet, and the name has become a trademark for a delicious dish that is now known all over the world. It is important that with the combination of oats and milk Bircher-Benner found a protein-based combination, showing in its amino acid value a surplus of lysine, cystine and threonine, and thus equivalent in biological value to egg protein. The effect of a protein-based combination of oats and a little milk has since been confirmed by Professor J. Kühnau and Dr Wendel Gansmann.[1]

## REFINED FOODS

The consumer calls the tune, and consumers tend to be lured not by nutritive value but by appearance. The housewife likes the look of the pure white flour she uses to make her cakes, thicken her sauces, coat the fish she is going to fry. She lets the shiny white rice run through her

[1]*Oats: an element in modern nutrition*, Umschau-Verlag, Frankfurt-am-Main, 1976.

fingers. She sprinkles snowy white sugar over the fruit salad. She slices the soft white bread. What she does not realise is that the 'purity' she welcomes from her grocer and baker has been achieved industrially by refining operations and chemical whitening agents, all of which are toxic to some degree. The danger may seem slight – and so it would be if one only ate, say, one small loaf of bread per month, and did not use sugar or a whole host of other foods that have either been refined or discoloured and then recoloured (like oil or butter). They cause a slow build-up of poisons in our systems, which is dangerous precisely because it is not apparent at first.

More important, perhaps, is the fact that products thus denatured become dead – foods that cannot enhance life or health. In white rice, for instance, all that is left is starch. When milk has lost its whey and buttermilk, a lot of its nutritive value has gone. The life-giving essence of the oleaginous seeds from which our cooking oils are made goes into cattle-cake, to help stimulate milk production, rather than into nourishing us. Whole natural oil of first extraction that has not been exposed to heat is the only sort that retains its value.

But it is probably bread, such a staple part of our diet, that suffers most from the refining process. Public opinion has been built up over many years to believe that white bread is the accepted norm because coarse wholewheat bread used to be the food of the poor, while the rich could enjoy its soft, white counterpart. Then, during the nineteenth century, there was a great change in eating habits. To stimulate and expand the sale of manufactured products by pleasing the consumer, flour and sugar began to be whitened industrially, which meant that working people could also afford white sugar and flour. The poor thus felt they were eating the food of the rich. (The processing of oils and dairy products began later, though for different psychological reasons.) The new white flour and sugar were then saved for special occasions; they symbolised everything that was easy and luxurious. In fact, there was a French saying, 'Manger son pain blanc en premier', which meant 'Getting off to a good start'. Today, unfortunately, many people eat *only* white bread. And that is not even made of pure wheat, for it is permitted to add a certain proportion of rice-flour (to make it whiter still) and starch, while the most valuable element in the wheat – the wheatgerm – is removed. It is impossible to overstress the importance of changing to wholemeal bread – either wheat or rye (the latter being advisable in cases of intestinal sluggishness).

Experiments carried out in some hospital gastroenterology departments, in which patients were given only wholemeal bread, produced such conclusive results that this became regular practice.

One of Max Bircher-Benner's theories (still being researched) was that food should be eaten whole, with none of its components removed. Milk that has had the cream removed to make butter, for instance, is no longer a whole food. As he put it: 'The harmonious balance of all the parts which occurs in natural foodstuffs cannot be improved upon at will, but is in fact more likely to be destroyed by any interference. Not even the most "scientific" processes can then re-create it ...'

Only whole foods contain the principles of life: the processed versions do not make adequate substitutes.

# 6. Stimulants

Whatever the complaint being treated, Max Bircher-Benner categorically banned all stimulants from his diets and treatments: all alcohol, tobacco, coffee, tea.

They are called stimulants because they have the effect of spurring us on, giving our flagging systems that slight stimulus, that illusion of well-being, that enables us to go on driving our bodies when they would naturally be demanding a rest. Stimulants are thus not only dangerous for the harm they themselves do, but also for the way they temporarily mask their destructive action, preventing our becoming aware of fatigue, which is always a warning sign. Once we become used to taking stimulants, they rapidly develop into a need. The small quantity that was enough at first soon becomes ineffective, so we take more, and by the time the danger is recognised, it is too late to stop. Indeed, serious direct effects, such as arterial disease, can occur without any warning if the dangers of taking stimulants are not appreciated.

One, two, three, four, six cups of coffee; a single whisky, drunk on the grounds that 'It is good for the heart, it's a vasodilator, my doctor says it's okay'. Can any doctor be so foolish? One drink follows another – and it's the same with cigarettes. Other people prefer tea as their pick-me-up; it is less dangerous, they say. Some people make no such distinction, and cheerfully ingest all these poisons. The nervous system cannot be driven on like this – once, ten times, a hundred times a day – with impunity. It pays the price in physical or mental illness.

It is important to grasp the fact that a need for such 'aids' is an indication of a weakness in the system. Rather than stimulating it artificially, we should be bracing and restoring it. People should be made aware that the human body has its own capacity for self-regeneration, and that the continuous and massive use of artificial stimulants actually works against the natural regeneration essential to health.

The Bircher-Benner system of diet rejects all artificial methods of stimulating the sympathetic nervous system, in favour of letting the natural regenerating action of the parasympathetic system operate. Only thus can the body achieve optimum efficiency, and so be able to overcome infections and illness by a build-up of natural resistance.

A slightly less dangerous temporary boost comes from sweets, candies, chocolate, all of which cause sugar to be pumped into the bloodstream, giving a quick spurt of energy. Though not so poisonous, they have harmful effects on the liver, the veins and the heart, and contribute to poor nutrition, vascular disease and obesity.

## MEAT

People would not usually think of adding meat to their list of stimulants, yet it belongs there for four reasons: first, because of its excess of proteins; second, because of its uric acid content; third, because of the extracts found in the broth when it is stewed; and fourth, because of the substances produced by sudden exposure to violent heat, as when meat is grilled.

Initially, Bircher-Benner included meat in his system of nutrition but as time went on his experiments and research led him to exclude it. We, his children, grew up without ever eating meat, and our growth never suffered for lack of it. I used to hear people talking about delicious roasts, or superb new meat dishes they had enjoyed, and one day I asked my father what this apparently wonderful food was like. He always preferred persuasion to prohibition, knowing that forbidden fruit would always retain its magic, and that only discipline that was freely accepted could be effective. So before lunch the next day he presented me with a nice little parcel – of red meat. I was appalled: was this what people ate? My father insisted that it be cooked in the normal way, and made me eat some of it. It remains one of my most unpleasant memories.

However, though meat was excluded from all Bircher-Benner cures and strict diets, he never forbade his patients to eat it in moderation. The same applied to fish, so long as it was eaten near where it was caught, so that it was absolutely fresh. But, since he saw no special nutritional value in meat that could not be found in dairy products, cereals, nuts, dried fruits, and fresh fruit and vegetables, he never included it in his approved diets. Furthermore, though his attitude to meat was relatively flexible, he would allow no compromise where offal was concerned, especially kidneys and liver (the only permissible item was heart, a muscle). These filtering organs were, by their nature, full of uric acid and toxic waste products of all kinds and must never be eaten. (How much more strongly would he say this today, with all the hormones and various poisonous substances that are now used in the forced feeding of animals!)

In general, however, Bircher-Benner was always prepared to allow exceptions to his rules – provided they remained the exception. He did not think some unhealthy food would lead to disease, unless the unhealthy eating pattern had become a habit that was out of control.

Protein, of course, is essential to life, building up the tissue of muscles and nerves, bones and cartilage. But, whereas it used to be believed in Bircher-Benner's day that protein meant animal protein and, more recently, that one could hardly have too much protein, and that at least one-third of one's food should be of animal origin, it has now been accepted that Bircher-Benner was right in maintaining that 50g (2 oz) of protein a day is adequate for a person weighing 70kg (150 lb). Recent international gerontology congresses have endorsed this view, and have also confirmed that the protein in green vegetables and whole cereals – especially in combination – is of a higher biological quality than protein of animal origin, and therefore has more nutritive value.

In fact, at the last Congress of the World Food and Agriculture Organisation a strong recommendation was issued that we should reduce our consumption of animal protein by a third. And recently another eminent pioneer in the field of dietetics, Professor Lothar Wendt, has demonstrated that deposits on the capillaries caused by an excess of animal protein are responsible for much of the contemporary prevalence of degenerative diseases.[1] A revolution indeed – but one that Max Bircher-Benner was calling for three-quarters of a century earlier. Unfortunately, success in persuading people to change to healthier eating habits has not been in proportion to the efforts made. Indeed, a contemporary of Dr Bircher-Benner's, Professor Emil Terroine, wrote as early as 1933: 'Some strange instinct seems to drive us to avoid what is best in every group of foodstuffs, and the most valuable elements in everything nature produces.'[2]

[1] *Krankheiten verminderter Kapillarmembran Permeabilität,* by Professor Lothar Wendt, of the Johann Wolfgang Goethe University, Frankfurt (Verlag E. E. Koch, Frankfurt, 1974–6).
[2] *Metabolisme de l'Azote,* by Professor Emil F. Terroine, of the University of Strasbourg (Presses Universitaires de France, Paris, 1933), p. 247.

# 7. The Order of Life

'What we have to cure sickness with is life' – the entire teaching of Max Bircher-Benner can be summed up in those words. Though he made his own the famous statement of the Japanese nutritionist, Dr Katase, 'Diet is the sovereign mistress of life and health',[1] he did not use his newly discovered treatment of raw foods in isolation. He sought to draw strength from those other sources of life – air, sun and water.

## AIR

Patients were surprised to find 'air-bathing' listed at the end of the prescriptions Bircher-Benner handed to them. But, as he explained to them, 'Normally only the skin of your face and hands breathes. You are depriving your body of the vital function of breathing through all its pores.' They were to take 'baths' in the fresh air, in the shade if it was not too cold, and if possible they should only wear a bathing suit so that their bodies were well exposed to the air. People who lived in town, without a garden or access to the countryside, could take air-baths by an open window quite beneficially. A half-hour (or even a quarter) of exercises, followed by ten minutes' air-bathing, is a tremendous tonic. Bircher-Benner considered such air-baths – for up to an hour – good for the skin, the heart, the circulation, and the whole respiratory system. He knew that people must learn to breathe properly, and get the air circulating both internally and externally. Could there be any better way of 'scouring out' the lungs, of regularising

[1] *Der Einfluss der Ernährung auf die Konstitution des Organismus* (Verlag Urban und Schwarzenberg, Berlin, 1934).

65

the heartbeat, of getting the whole neuro-vegetative system back into balance? Emptying the lungs and emptying the mind – for you cannot think when your whole body is involved in breathing properly – is a vital aid to health.

## SUN

Bircher-Benner advocated various forms of contact with nature. At a date when people still feared exposure to the sun, he attributed great importance to its effects, which a few enterprising doctors were beginning to investigate. He realised that the light, heat and chemical action of the sun's rays had various effects on the tissues – germicidal, anti-inflammatory, healing, analgesic and stimulating (increasing the red blood-cells). Though he never saw the ravages that were to be caused in later years by prolonged and unregulated sunbathing (burns, dry skin, acute or chronic skin conditions, pulmonary and circulatory lesions, heat stroke, and so on) he strictly limited the time his patients spent in the sun: ten minutes at first, increasing gradually by five minutes a day to a maximum of an hour. He considered that a successful treatment was one that produced a golden tan, leaving the skin soft and supple, thus indicating that the patient was reacting properly to the ultra-violet rays. When the skin could not tolerate sun and became red in patches instead of producing an even pigmentation, it indicated, among other things, poor circulation and a tendency to congestion. No indication of this kind ever escaped his notice.

To the dry heat of the sun he attributed analgesic and curative powers of particular value to sufferers from rheumatic and arthritic ailments. Therefore, when circumstances made sunbathing impossible, or the patient could not tolerate it, he substituted a sun lamp, to be used in the bedroom when resting and relaxing (see the appendix on Types of Treatment).

## WATER: HYDROTHERAPY

The third element, water, is vital to the Bircher system: indeed, the ways in which he used it made it appear almost miraculous. I can best illustrate this by some personal memories.

One day, long before the advent of antibiotics, one of my friends came to me in great distress to tell me that her little brother was seriously ill: he had a boil on his upper lip, and the doctor, seeing that the infection was spreading over his face, had declared that there was nothing he could do for him. I rushed into my father's study and told him about it. As usual, his response was instantaneous: he took us to the car, and within minutes we were at the child's bedside. He lay there, his face swollen and inflamed, his eyes almost shut, with a temperature of 40°C (104°F). He could barely whimper. My father told me later that at that moment he had given him up for lost, but he picked up the hot little body, and asked to be shown the bathroom. There he turned on the cold tap, and ran it gently on to the boil for a minute. He told the mother to do the same thing for precisely a minute every hour.

It seemed hardly credible that a child whose life was despaired of could be saved by a little water – but hope is powerful, and my father possessed great authority. The mother obeyed, and the following day the crisis was over; within a few days the child was fully recovered.

Cold water is effective wherever there is inflammation – in mastoid infections, phlebitis, and so on. The body's reaction to cold water involves a contraction and dilation of the blood vessels and capillaries, which stimulates the circulation, thereby providing more white blood cells to attack and destroy toxins. So the child had been saved by a completely natural process.

Equally spectacular, and perhaps even more incredible, was a case that happened in about 1935. A family of friends from Alsace used to spend their holidays in their country house outside Zurich. One morning, one of their five children woke up complaining of a headache. His mother took little notice, but as the day wore on it grew worse, and by the evening the child showed signs of paralysis. Her first thought was that it must be poliomyelitis, for which there was no vaccine in those days. She had no car, and there was no telephone. Zurich was more than thirty miles away, and she knew that speed was vital. The child was crying, and complaining that he could not breathe. She soaked a sheet in cold water, and wrapped his body in it, with wool blankets outside. She prepared a second sheet and, as soon as the first was warm, she replaced it, and continued changing the sheets all night. She thought she noticed a slight improvement the next morning, but at the end of forty-eight hours she was exhausted, and had begun to doubt whether there was any point in going on. However, in the night of the third day, the little boy moved – first an arm, then a leg. She took his temperature, and found that the fever had gone. The child recovered.

This woman had been brought up on my father's principles, and had remembered his saying that if a child had a high fever and symptoms of paralysis, he must be wrapped in cold sheets without a moment's delay. (See 'Priessnitz packs' in the appendix on Types of Treatment.)

Another story comes from my cousin, Dr Dagmar Liechti von Brasch:

I was twenty-four, and in my second year as an intern. I was perfectly healthy generally, but I caught influenza (viral, probably) and while I was recovering from that I woke up one day to find that half my face was paralysed. I could not close my left eye, part of my tongue was numb, and I'd partially lost my sense of smell. My first reaction was one of amusement – I looked comical in the extreme. But by the end of three days it seemed less funny, for the paralysis was spreading to the right side, and my face was a horrible sight. I immediately thought of my uncle. But, though we all loved and respected him, we were afraid of him, too, and I didn't feel I could bother him just for myself. I went to see Dr V., our ear, nose and throat professor, and asked his advice. He examined me thoroughly, then told me how sorry he was to have to give a colleague such a bad prognosis.

'This sort of facial paralysis is very likely to persist and become chronic, because the damage to the facial nerve is irreversible. With luck there could be a slight improvement in six weeks or so, but I'm very much afraid that you'll have to learn to live with the semi-paralysis. The only advice I can give', he added, with a wry smile, 'is to make sure you don't catch another cold.'

I was appalled, and the more I looked in the mirror the worse I felt. What sort of life could I look forward to with a face like that? I no longer had any compunction about disturbing my uncle.

He also examined me carefully, but not only my face. He went over my entire body – skin, reflexes, temperature, blood pressure, blood tests, everything. Then he said:

'You'll get better, but you are going to need a lot of energy – the treatment will require the most rigid discipline.'

What he prescribed was two weeks in bed on a diet of raw vegetables only, an hour's sweating a day, Priessnitz (cold) packs, and electrical galvanisation of the affected facial nerve. I was to have no visitors, and to speak only when absolutely necessary; to be as calm as possible and try not to worry too much.

Chewing raw vegetables on one side of my mouth was extremely difficult. The sweating, followed by cold packs, was extremely unpleasant. Then, just as I was relaxed and going peacefully to sleep, they gave me galvanic shocks. But on the fourth day I felt the muscles on my left side moving a little. I found I could taste some of the herbs in my food, and I could actually shut my left eye. I could have cried for joy. By the seventh day, my face was moving normally.

I had a further week's treatment, and then, looking like my normal self, went back to work. My colleagues were astounded.

Wonderful, perhaps, but there was nothing miraculous about this cure. The causes of a paralysis of the facial nerve can be various – poliomyelitis, a virus infection; a chill causing the tunnel containing the nerve to swell, thus compressing the nerve itself. In my cousin's case it was the latter. Unfortunately, there is a danger that the compressed nerve will be permanently damaged, and this was what Professor V. thought had happened. But my father had the most profound reluctance to accept anything as irreversible; his faith in nature was total, and he truly believed what we all say so lightly: 'While there's life, there's hope.' So he applied a kind of shock treatment, to attack from all sides at once:

1  raw vegetables, without salt, low in protein, rich in potassium, to help get rid of the swelling;

2  vitamins B and C contained in the raw vegetables, to increase resistance to the virus;

3  sweating, to get rid of toxins, while at the same time raising the temperature artificially and thus creating an effective defensive reaction;

4 galvanisation or shock treatment: interstitial electrolysis to act on the paralysed muscle and nerve, causing artificial movement;

5 cold packs, to stimulate the whole circulatory system, relaxing and contracting nerves and muscles. Their calming effect is crucial in any ailment where the nerves play so large a part.

In this particular case, the Bircher-Benner treatment was to have a far greater effect on his niece than just curing her facial paralysis. 'For years afterwards,' she says, 'I did not have a single catarrhal ailment or influenza. My health had never been so good. And I had also undergone a profound physical and emotional experience – I became aware, as never before, of the curative powers of nature.'

## THE ORDER OF LIFE

Max Bircher-Benner's philosophy – his spiritual teaching, if you like – can be summed up as 'respecting the order of life, and being in harmony with oneself'. When he asked that same niece to go to London in his place, to treat a famous psychotherapist, and she felt the responsibility was too great, he simply wrote, 'Do what you think best, and you'll do the right thing.' And once, when she was concerned over the best treatment for someone, he replied, 'To cure anyone there must be a harmonious co-operation between the patient, the doctor – and God.' He had a wisdom that grew out of deep study and research. He considered that the order of life was continually being interfered with and the balance destroyed; that we are part of a whole scheme of things and should be in harmony with it. His attitude to walking illustrates this point. To him walking had all the obvious health advantages, of course. It was good exercise, good muscular activity, calming to the nerves; it assisted the circulation, increasing the pumping-power of the heart, dilating the arteries, increasing the blood supply to the veins and thus increasing the oxygen supply and removing the most deep-seated impurities from the respiratory system. But it was also the finest way for human beings to be really in touch with nature.

To be aware of one's environment is the first step: to admire, value and love nature is the basis of understanding it, and understanding nature shows us the way towards rediscovering our own biological balance – the way our bodies really work. Ralph Bircher, one of his sons, often used to say that everything was regulated by a kind of 'biological clock'. These inner rhythms can be seen as being in relation with the astronomic rhythm of the sun, the gravitational system of our own planet, with the alternation of light and darkness – hence the importance of not confusing day and night, of not destroying the cosmic rhythm. (Dr Bircher-Benner always insisted that the sleep of the hours before midnight was the most restorative, and his clinic has always been run on this principle.)

Respecting the order of life in diet as well as routine, in work as well as amusements, not going against nature or forcing it, being in harmony with one's own deepest self, were Max Bircher-Benner's rules of life.

I can see him now, at the end of his life, working in his study with its gleaming dark furniture, the walls covered in bookshelves, his back to the large window that looked out on to the snow-clad park. There he wrote articles and letters or worked on his notes. He had a great deal of perspicacity. He could not be deceived, by other people, by his scientific colleagues, or by his old enemy, disease. When he was dying, he knew it.

The beard sweeping down over his collar was completely white, his receding hair made his forehead larger. Hollows beneath the skin made the fine bone-structure stand out. He sighed not because he was leaving life – that he knew was inevitable, and he had long been prepared for it – but because there was still so much to be done. He sighed because, although he had turned his body into a strong and resilient tool despite the initial handicap of a premature birth, he could do nothing to overcome the weakness of his heart. He could perhaps have spared himself more – but that would have meant at least partly reducing his work, which was unthinkable. Many would have taken to their beds, but he was determined to remain up, and he only went to bed for the final weeks, after a violent heart attack.

I had always been very close to him and visited him daily, and my cousin, his pupil, Dr. Liechti von Brasch, who he so much hoped would continue his work in the future, gave him medical care. He could look back over his life with some contentment: his sons were doctors or economists, his daughters were happily married, his wife was with him, loving and attentive. There was peace in the thought that his work as a man had been a success. His work as a doctor was unfinished – but others would follow him, and others would follow them; one day, the work might possibly be finished.

Even in bed he put on his glasses again and took up his pen. He still hoped to complete the work he was writing on the diet of the Hunzas, whose way of life and excellent physique were living proof of the value of his own ideas.[1] On 24 January 1939, from his bed, my father dictated to his secretary the final pages of his book. It was 'The End' in every sense. He was seventy-two.

But, though the man was dead, his work lived on. The clinic continued to exist under the auspices of his two sons,

---

[1]Since then, our civilisation has overtaken them, and given them the same diseases as the rest of us.

Doctors Willy and Franklin Bircher, and his niece, Doctor Dagmar Liechti. Four years later, I gave up my career as a violinist to become administrative director of the clinic that had meant so much to my father.

On 15 November 1967, the centenary of Max Bircher-Benner's birth, 250 doctors and professors from all over the world came to Zurich to honour the memory of the man who founded the modern science of dietetics. Professor Alfred Gigon, of Basle, President of the Swiss Academy of Medical Sciences, concluded his speech with a quotation from Plutarch: 'It is by remembering great men and great works that the present is linked to the past and makes ready for the future.'

# 8. Health at the Meal Table

To follow Dr Bircher-Benner's rules of diet is to make health a guest at your table. But to derive the best advantage from them – to feel better, and live better – you must observe certain elementary but vital principles.

## PLANNING THE ORDER

It is not enough simply to lay out a dish of raw vegetables, a bowl of muesli or other cereals, and a chunk of brown bread. The meal must be properly planned. The succession of dishes matters: you cannot eat just anything in just any order.

The effectiveness of raw foods is increased if they are eaten at the beginning of the meal, because of the curious phenomenon of digestive leucocytosis. It has been observed that the moment the first mouthful of any cooked or processed food is swallowed, a mass of white corpuscles appears on the intestinal wall. They remain there for between an hour and an hour and a half, and constitute a massive mobilisation of defences against the food that is being eaten (the role of white blood-cells is to fight infection). The process is completely normal, but what is surprising is that it does not happen with raw food. It was this phenomenon, combined with other chemical processes, that made Dr Bircher-Benner recommend starting a meal with fresh fruit, and following that with a green salad, in order to prevent this wasted expenditure of white blood-cells.

Why should a green salad follow the fruit? Green leaves are so rich in vitamins, mineral salts and protein – and these are present in such perfect proportions – that they should be our first priority. Even traditional medicine recommends that those suffering from gastric ulcers start their meals with a green vegetable.

Professor W. Schuphan,[1] a recognised authority on nutrition, writes that 'green leaves in addition provide nutritive substances that are of fundamental importance, qualitatively and quantitatively, for the diet of both people and animals'. This is nowadays universally recognised. Leafy vegetables are thus more valuable than any others. There is, for example, as much lysine in 272g of broccoli as in an ordinary egg.[2] The cabbage family in general ranks high, its different varieties offering an exceptional range of nutrients. Its green leaves are of special biological value for their vitamin C and pro-vitamin A. The family includes kohlrabi, cauliflower, Brussels sprouts, and kale. Another leafy vegetable not yet well known in the West is Chinese cabbage: its proteins have great biological value, and it has high levels of mineral salts and vitamin C. Indeed, it has been found to supply so much protein that a Chinese vegetarian diet can consist of vegetables alone (though it is important to note that this is only satisfactory when every meal includes a sufficient variety of vegetables).

When planning what raw fruit and vegetables should appear on the table, you must obey a simple rule: a whole plant should be represented: leaf, stem, fruit and root. This does not mean serving carrots with their tops left on, but merely that a meal should contain all four elements. For instance the root may be carrots, the leaf and stem can be lettuce or spinach, the fruit tomato or whatever fruit is in season. This will provide the entire range of vitamins and mineral salts necessary to health.

[1] Of the University of Mainz; Director of the Geisenheim Institute of Agriculture.
[2] *Summary of Nutritive Values* by Drs Souci, Fachmann and Krauch (Stuttgart, 1969).

## HOW TO BEGIN

To adopt the Bircher-Benner dietary system means doing away with many years of cooking habits and inherited tastes; it also calls for a major psychological change. You cannot change your eating patterns overnight; to do that would almost certainly result in failure. Never try to give up your old ways all at once, but start at first with a short 'overhaul' period (see Detoxication, p. 127). Never start with a crash cure except on medical advice, especially if there is anything seriously wrong with you.

You must start in the right conditions – of time, of place, of intention. And you must be absolutely determined to stick to the number of days proposed – two weeks at least, preferably three. Attitude is also important: it is no good feeling that you might as well try this as anything else; it must be a serious undertaking.

Depending on the results achieved by the 'overhaul' period you might take one of several decisions: to repeat the cure at the beginning of every season, making a point of using the fruit and vegetables of the season in each case; or partially to adopt this form of diet while still keeping some of your old ways (though these must be strictly limited – no pork in any form, for instance, no offal, no butter in cooking, no sauces, no refined foods, no stimulants, and so on); or, if you feel the treatment has changed you completely, to switch to the Bircher-Benner system without a backward glance.

## LEARNING HOW TO EAT

Following such a diet does not mean renouncing the pleasures of the table. Quite the opposite, in fact. It means developing new tastes and enjoying food in a more subtle way. It is vitally important to eat with relish. Sitting down to a meal should never be a boring duty. The dishes served should be pleasing to the eye as well as the palate but, when offered new flavours, the palate may have to learn to enjoy them. As you grow older your sense of taste develops and changes. Alcohol and tobacco dull our appreciation of tastes. When you give a child wine for the first time, he makes a face. Children are always suspicious of strong, sharp, unfamiliar tastes; we all have to be educated to tolerate and then enjoy them. But is 'education' the right word? Surely, we in fact *pervert* our natural tastes? At first, without the seasoning we are used to, this new kind of food may strike us as tasteless; and the more we swallow it without chewing properly, the more its subtleties escape us. We have to give our taste buds time to get to know what we are eating.

Because the mouth is the first organ of digestion, its action governs and determines the entire process. Its role is to prepare food for digestion, with the help of the teeth, the saliva glands and the taste buds. When the mouth fails to do its job properly, the digestive function is upset – the root cause of a great many gastric and intestinal problems. If food is to be rushed through, it obviously has to be artificially and strongly seasoned in order to have any taste at all. We do not give our taste buds time to act reflexively on the nervous system, on the secretion of gastric juices, so that disorders of various kinds are bound to ensue.

Enjoyment starts when the food comes into contact with the mouth. Dr Bircher-Benner used to say that this was a vitally important action, an act of life that one should perform with due self-respect. There are a great many different flavours to be discovered in fruit, raw vegetables, the various leafy salads, and cereals – a variety to delight the most subtle of gourmets.

A further advantage of eating slowly is that it prevents overeating. People who overeat put unnecessary strain on their system and if energy-giving foods are not burnt off with extra activity they result in fat. Bircher-Benner said: 'Whatever we eat over and above our real needs weakens rather than fortifies us, contrary to accepted belief. In terms of genuine health it is a positive disadvantage. While it is true that good health demands a superabundance of life-giving substances, especially of vitamins and mineral salts, it only needs a limited quantity of energy-giving foods.' It is not the quantity we eat, but its quality, that nourishes us. Overeating is one of the gravest dangers to which we can subject our bodies. Current research has discredited the idea that for a human being to be healthy and strong he or she must be stuffed with food from the cradle to the grave, that not being overfed means being underfed.

A leading American nutritionist, Clive McCay,[1] of Cornell University, conducted an interesting experiment. He fed one lot of animals slightly less food than they could actually absorb, so that they had a mild sensation of hunger all the time. The quality of what they ate, however, was carefully monitored; they had various cereals and green vegetables. He gave a second lot whatever and as much as they wanted to eat. In the first lot as a result:

1 diseases of old age usual in the species disappeared;
2 their average lifespan increased considerably; and
3 they remained lively, in very good physical condition.
In the second lot precisely the opposite happened.

Professor Kutatsune of the University of Kyoto made what may perhaps be considered the most conclusive experiment. In 1951 he and his wife put themselves on a daily diet containing only the number of calories given in

[1] Professor McCay is an authority on diet and ageing. The experiment referred to here is described in his article 'The Effects of restricted feeding upon ageing and chronic diseases in rats and dogs', *American Journal of Public Health*, May 1947.

concentration camps, but in the form of raw vegetables, fruit and cereals. They were able to do their jobs as usual, without feeling hungry or unwell in any way. After three months of this, they changed to a diet containing the same number of calories, but in the form of conventional food. Within a month it looked as if they were becoming seriously ill and so they were forced to abandon the experiment.

The way we distribute our food over the day is also very important. More and more dieticians are recommending (even in slimming diets) that breakfast, the first meal after twelve hours without food, should be properly nourishing. The midday meal should restore us after a morning's work and prepare us for the rest of the day. In the evening, if we observe the rhythm of nature, we should go to bed early, so it is pointless to eat too large a meal – doing so may also cause insomnia.

Following these rules ensures that the cure is effective, for it depends not merely on turning to different food but on adopting a different pattern of life, in harmony with nature and your own being (bearing in mind that respecting nature also means respecting yourself and refusing to damage your body).

## CHOOSING AND PREPARING FRUIT AND VEGETABLES

If you have a garden, make the most of it by growing your own vegetables in the old-fashioned way, without using chemical fertilisers or poisons of any kind (slug pellets, caterpillar or aphid sprays, and so on). What kills small creatures rapidly will slowly but surely kill large ones too. City dwellers may not have the luxury of a vegetable garden. They must therefore find the shopkeeper who sells the freshest produce. If you are following a Bircher-Benner diet, you *must* eat organically-grown vegetables. Grown as our ancestors grew their food, they cost more than others, but they really are better, both in taste and in nutritional value. If you cannot shop regularly in a health-food shop or department, do at least buy your root vegetables there – potatoes, carrots, tubers of all kinds. The parts of plants exposed to the air and sun rid themselves more easily of the various fertilisers than those underground.

A really fresh vegetable should be firm and well-coloured (and some types, such as cucumber or aubergine, should gleam). Fruit should be ripe, but not bruised or over-ripe.

Don't trust fruit that is too beautiful, too symmetrical: nature seldom turns out such perfection unaided. It is a thousand times better to eat a small, local-grown apple than a large luscious-looking one from miles away.

Do not assume that as long as vegetables have been bought fresh they can be kept in the kitchen for five or six days before being eaten. They can be kept for a maximum of forty-eight hours, in the refrigerator (at 4–6°C or 39–43°F), wrapped in paper to prevent dehydration. If you grow your own, you can freeze them, but it is important to do this correctly, and the procedure varies from one vegetable to another. Incorrectly frozen vegetables may *taste* deliciously fresh three months later, but will have lost all their food value. Everything must be frozen in polythene containers labelled with the date. Vegetables must be thoroughly washed, cut into circles or cubes and blanched beforehand. A couple of centimetres' space should be left in the container for expansion. The vegetables should be eaten within three to four months.

Try not to prepare the whole day's supply of raw vegetables in the morning. From the time they are peeled, grated or chopped, living foods become vulnerable to oxygen and heat. Peeled fruits and vegetables can only be kept cooked if they are in a syrup or stock that protects them from the air.

Remember that it is the *green* leaves of vegetables like cabbage and lettuce that you should be keeping and eating for their carotene and albumin. White leaves, with no chlorophyll and very little taste, are far less valuable.

You should throw out the stalks of cultivated mushrooms, because they absorb chemicals from fertilisers; they should also be skinned just before eating, since contact with the air poisons the skin of the mushroom.

There are microbes in all fruit and vegetables, however healthy – even in those that have just been picked, let alone those that have been handled a lot before you get them. So they must always be washed, especially salad greens, in salt water (a handful of sea-salt to 5 litres of water). If they are very dirty, add a quarter of a glass of vinegar or a few drops of lemon juice (citric and acetic acid both have a powerful bactericidal effect).

If you live in a tropical climate there are further precautions you must take: soak all vegetables in a 5 per cent solution of permanganate, or in a chloride of lime solution (5g per litre of water). Place all roots and fruit-vegetables, such as tomatoes, in boiling water for ten seconds. Finally, always add one part lemon juice to four of other fruit or vegetable juices.

Your vegetables, now healthy, fresh and clean, must be made attractive to those who are to eat them. It is important to present them harmoniously – colour is important in the arrangement of food, and dishes that please the eye are far more appetising.

Never overcook vegetables: soup left simmering for a long time loses its vitamins and essential salts. Vegetables should not boil for more than twenty minutes, and it is preferable to steam them, as rapidly as possible. Except in cases of special sensitivity (of the mucous membrane, for example), food should not be reduced to a mush: vegetables should remain firm, almost crisp. Cut them into large chunks, so that they still have to be chewed – chewing is an important factor in the digestive process.

Add parsley, mint, chives, basil or other chopped herbs to your dishes. They add attractive colour and flavour to the vegetables, and also contribute large amounts of vitamins and mineral salts. Parsley and chervil are particularly rich in iron. (See Seasonings, p. 101.)

## Suggestions for Preparing Raw Vegetables and Salads

### Mixed Salads

| | | |
|---|---|---|
| Chicory and diced tomatoes | Oil dressing | Garlic |
| Green peppers and fennel | Oil dressing | |
| Fennel, chicory and diced tomatoes | Mayonnaise | |
| Fennel and carrots | Cream dressing | |
| Tomatoes and green peppers | Oil dressing or mayonnaise | |

### Stuffing for Tomatoes

| | |
|---|---|
| Cucumber | Oil dressing or mayonnaise |
| Celery | Cream dressing |
| Cauliflower | Cream dressing |
| White cabbage | Mayonnaise |

(Chives, parsley and onion can be added in small quantities to all raw vegetables.)

## Suggestions for Preparing Raw Vegetables and Salads

| Type of salad | Preparation | Dressing | Seasoning |
|---|---|---|---|
| Lettuce | Uncut | Oil dressing (oil and lemon juice) | Chives, onion |
| Lettuce | Cut into 1 cm (half-inch) strips | Oil dressing or mayonnaise | Basil, marjoram |
| Lamb's lettuce | Uncut | Oil dressing | Chives, onion |
| Endive | Cut into 1 cm (half-inch) strips | Oil dressing or mayonnaise | Chives, onion, parsley |
| Watercress | Uncut | Oil dressing or mayonnaise | Onion |
| Spinach | Cut into 1 cm (half-inch) strips | Oil dressing or mayonnaise | Mint |
| Cabbage salad (white cabbage, sauerkraut, Brussels sprouts, kale) | Shred finely | Oil dressing or mayonnaise | Lovage, thyme, cumin, savory |
| Tomatoes | Cut in half or slice | Oil dressing or mayonnaise | Basil, thyme, dill |
| Cucumber | Slice very finely | Oil dressing or mayonnaise | Dill |
| Fennel | Cut coarsely or chop finely | Oil dressing or mayonnaise | Onion, chives |
| Green peppers | Cut into strips | Oil dressing | Chives |
| Horseradish | Mince or grate | Oil or cream dressing | Chives |

| Radishes | Grate | Oil or cream dressing | Chives |
|---|---|---|---|
| Celery | Slice finely | Oil or cream dressing | Onion, chives |
| Courgettes (or zucchini) | Cut in strips or chop coarsely | Oil dressing or mayonnaise | Dill, borage, basil |
| Carrots | Grate finely | Cream or oil dressing | Marjoram, lovage |
| Celeriac | Grate finely | Cream or oil dressing | Basil, thyme |
| Beetroot | Grate | Cream dressing or mayonnaise | Lovage, thyme, cumin |
| Cauliflower | Grate the stalk | Cream dressing or mayonnaise | Basil, marjoram, walnuts |
| Chicory | Cut into 1 cm (half-inch) strips | Cream or oil dressing | Tarragon, marjoram |
| Jerusalem artichokes | Grate | Cream dressing | Thyme, balm |
| Kohlrabi | Shred and mince or chop very small | Cream or oil dressing | Thyme, lovage |
| Red cabbage | Shred or chop finely | Cream or oil dressing | A little grated apple, cumin, lovage |

# 9. Food Fit for a Gourmet

Following a diet does not mean that you can no longer enjoy food – eating should still remain one of life's pleasures. The recipes given in this chapter are just some examples of the variety that can be introduced into the Bircher-Benner diet. You can use them as a basis for introducing your own ideas, provided you stick to the principles.[1]

## SALADS

### Celeriac
Take a celeriac weighing about ½ kg (1 lb), and cut it into matchsticks. Add 1 tablespoonful of lemon juice, 6 roughly-chopped walnuts, a grated apple and a pinch of salt. Dress with soya-flour mayonnaise (see p. 87), to which may be added (if you are greedy and your digestion is good) two tablespoonfuls of cream.

### Sauerkraut
Shake and rinse the sauerkraut. To each 100g (4 oz) sauerkraut, add a finely-chopped onion and an apple cut into fine strips. Mix with some cumin seed (or ground cumin) and a few juniper berries. Pour over, drop by drop, the juice of a lemon and two tablespoonfuls of pure olive oil (first cold-press extraction).

### Cabbage and sauerkraut salad
This may be made with equal quantities of sauerkraut,

[1]See *Livre de cuisine Bircher-Benner* (Editions Bircher-Benner, Bad Homburg vor der Höhe, and Zürich Erlenbach). Available in English: *Eating Your Way to Health*, by Ruth Bircher, translated and edited by Claire Loewenfeld (Faber, London, 1961).

shredded Brussels sprouts and Chinese cabbage (or red cabbage). Season with yoghourt dressing and chopped parsley. This is an unusual and very refreshing salad.

## Raw cabbage (Coleslaw)
Chop white cabbage into fine strips. Season with lemon juice and cumin.

## Cooked vegetable salad
Carrots, celery, celeriac, beans, and courgettes are all excellent to use cooked in salads. Dress with a French dressing consisting of 1 teaspoonful of lemon juice to each tablespoonful of olive oil (or any other oil you find digestible, except ground-nut oil) and some finely chopped herbs.

## Courgette salad
Slice firm courgettes into very fine rounds (like cucumber). Dress with soya-flour mayonnaise.

# DRESSINGS

Everyone is familiar with vinaigrette sauce (or French dressing) and mayonnaise. But there are alternatives which, though planned for special diets, are equally delicious.

## Cream dressing
2 parts of cream to 1 of low-fat soft cheese. Beat well together, adding lemon juice to taste, a little onion, and some chopped herbs.

## Soya-flour mayonnaise (for albumin-free diets)
2 tablespoonfuls of soya flour to 6 of water. Mix until smooth. Then slowly add 200ml (7 oz) pure olive oil and a

few drops of lemon juice, beating as for egg mayonnaise.

**Almond purée dressing (for albumin-free diets)**
3 parts of water to 1 of almond purée. Add lemon juice to
taste, and finely-chopped herbs. Mix thoroughly.

**Yoghourt dressing (for low-fat diets)**
1 teaspoonful of lemon juice to every 3 tablespoonfuls of
yoghourt. Mix with egg-whisk or in blender, and add
finely-chopped herbs.

## MUESLI

Muesli is a living food, and must therefore be eaten as soon
as it has been prepared. Any cereals may be used, though
oatmeal is traditionally the favourite. For variety you can
try mixing a teaspoon of oats with one of ground cereals
(wheat, rice, barley, rye, millet, buckwheat, or soya), and
mixing in some yeast flakes (vitamin B). The fruit should
be entirely untreated, and only juicy and moderately sour
apples chosen (do not use Golden Delicious, the production of which is too industrialised, or excessively acid green
apples). Sweetened condensed milk, which keeps many of
its biological qualities, is convenient, because you can use a
little at a time and it keeps. Substitute raw milk, if you
know a reliable supplier; or yoghourt. If sugar is used, it
must be unrefined cane sugar; if honey, it must be pure,
with no added sugar. Make sure the nuts added are fresh
and in good condition.
    It should be borne in mind that muesli is a light dish in
which fruit predominates over whatever cereal is used.

**MUESLI RECIPES (quantities for one serving)**

**Basic recipe**
8g (1 level tablespoon) oats
3 tablespoons water
1 tablespoon lemon juice
1 tablespoon sweetened condensed milk
200g (7 oz) apple
1 tablespoon grated hazelnuts or almonds
Soak the oats for 12 hours. (If using flaked or rolled oats, do not soak, but add the same quantity of water.) Add the lemon juice and milk. Stir until well mixed. Wash the apples and dry well with a clean towel. Remove the stalks, but leave the skins and cores. Grate directly into the mixture with a coarse grater (the apple must not be reduced to mush). Stir continuously to prevent the apple going brown. Sprinkle the nuts on top just before serving.

**Muesli with almond, hazelnut or sesame-seed purée**
(recommended in cases of allergy to animal protein)
8g (1 level tablespoon) oats
3 tablespoons water
1 tablespoon lemon juice
1 tablespoon almond, hazelnut or sesame-seed purée
1 tablespoon honey or unrefined dark cane sugar
3 tablespoons water (to replace the milk)
200g (7 oz) grated apple
1 tablespoon grated hazelnuts or almonds
Prepare as in the basic recipe above.

**Muesli with yoghourt**
(recommended in slimming diets, and for those who cannot tolerate milk)
8g (1 level tablespoon) oats
3 tablespoons water

3 tablespoons yoghourt
1 tablespoon lemon juice
1 tablespoon honey, or unrefined dark cane sugar
200g (7 oz) grated apple
1 tablespoon grated hazelnuts or almonds
Prepare as in the basic recipe above, making sure that the
yoghourt is smooth before adding it.

## Muesli with cream
(recommended for those who want to put on weight)
8g (1 tablespoon) oats
1–2 tablespoons water
3–4 tablespoons cream
1 teaspoon lemon juice
1 tablespoon honey
200g (7 oz) grated apple
1 tablespoon grated hazelnuts or almonds
Prepare as in the basic recipe above, whipping cream
lightly and mixing it with the lemon juice.

In all these recipes, small quantities of other raw fruit,
such as strawberries, raspberries, bilberries, bananas,
peaches, oranges, or mandarins, can be included as well as
the apple.

## Muesli for a diabetic diet
1g (¼–½ teaspoon) fresh barley-germ (see p. 91)
3g (1 teaspoon) soya sprouts (see p. 92)
4g (½ tablespoon) oats
3–4 tablespoons unsweetened evaporated milk
1–2 tablespoons water
1 tablespoon lemon juice
200g (7 oz) apple
1 tablespoon fructose syrup
1 tablespoon grated hazelnuts or almonds

Mix the barley-germ, soya sprouts and milk. Grate the apple and add with lemon juice to the water. Mix thoroughly. Add the fructose syrup, and sprinkle the nuts on top.

**Muesli with berries or soft fruit**
(especially rich in vitamin C)
The ingredients are the same as in the basic recipe above, but instead of the apple use 150–200g (5–7 oz) of one of the following: strawberries, raspberries, bilberries, redcurrants, blackberries, plums, peaches, or apricots. Prepare as in the basic recipe. If berries are used, they should be crushed with a pestle or mashed with a fork. Stone-fruits should be milled or chopped with a knife. In cases of gastro-intestinal disturbance, apricots and plums should be avoided.

## CEREAL DISHES

**Raw cereal: wheat, rye, oats or barley**
Wash the cereal grains and grind them quickly (in a coffee-mill or blender) to a coarse, flaky consistency. For each person mix 4–5 tablespoonfuls with 6–7 tablespoonfuls of water (do not use milk). Leave to soak overnight. Then add a helping of grated or finely chopped raw vegetables such as carrot, cucumber or tomato, or some raw fruit and a few drops of lemon juice or honey.

**Cooked cereal: wheat, rye, oats or barley**
Prepare cereal as above, and boil it in milk, or half milk and half water, to a medium consistency (not too smooth). Then, according to taste, add stewed or fresh fruit, cinnamon, brown sugar, or honey.

**Germinated grains and pulses**
During the process of germination, the protein in the

seeds of pulses (such as soya beans) and cereals becomes enriched with certain extremely active amino-acids, and produces large amounts of vitamins A and C. They also become very digestible and develop a pleasant, slightly sweet taste. They can be bought in health-food shops, but can easily be prepared at home:

*Preparation of germinated grains*
Soak the grains in twice their volume of water for 36 hours, leaving them in a cool dark room (15–18°C or 59–64°F). When they have absorbed all the water, spread out on a piece of cloth, and leave in the light in a warmer room (20–22°C, 68–72°F) for 3–5 days. By then sprouts and rootlets will have appeared, and the germinated grains can be eaten – either as they are or chopped and mixed with milk and sweetened, if possible, with honey. They can also be used in place of oats in muesli.

**Purée of cereals**
2 tablespoons cereals (wheat, oats, rye)
3 tablespoons water
Soak for 12 hours, then cook over a low heat for 10 minutes.

**Rice or barley water**
1 teaspoon rice or barley
200ml (7 oz) cold water
Cook for 5 minutes, stirring constantly. This may be added to fruit or vegetable juice in a proportion of 1 part of rice or barley water to 2 parts of juice.

**Linseed purée**
1 tablespoon linseed
200ml (7 oz) water
Wash the linseed well, mix with water and cook for 20

minutes. Strain. This may be added to juices, and is very helpful for cases of cystitis.

### Semolina
50g (scant 2 oz) semolina
500ml (17–18 oz) milk diluted with water
Sprinkle the semolina into boiling liquid, and cook for about 15 minutes, stirring constantly. You can add garlic and a bay-leaf before cooking; or, for a sweet dish, add, after cooking, 1 tablespoon sugar, 10g (¼–½ oz) butter, and sprinkle with cinnamon.

### Polenta
150g (5–6 oz) polenta (corn-meal)
1 litre (1¾ pint) water
salt
Sprinkle the polenta into boiling salted water, and cook gently for 20–40 minutes. Just before serving add, stirring constantly, 2 tablespoons grated cheese and a nut of butter.

## SOUPS

### Vegetable bouillon
All vegetables can be used to make excellent bouillon – not merely, as one might be led to believe, the regulation leeks, carrots and turnip. But remember that most vegetables should be washed only and not peeled.
1 onion
2 carrots
1 small head of celery
½ a Savoy cabbage
Few leaves spinach or spinach-beet
2 leeks
Bay-leaf, pinch of basil

Chop the vegetables up small. Bring to the boil in 2–3 litres (4–5 pints) cold water, and simmer over a low heat for 2 hours to extract all the flavour and food value. Strain off the bouillon, which can then be used as a basis for a great variety of soups. Here are four suggestions:

**Herb soup**
Mix 1 tablespoon flour (or cornflour) with a little cold milk till smooth, then pour into ½ litre (1 pt) boiling bouillon, stirring constantly. Season with basil, tarragon, marjoram, chives, parsley, and, if liked, a pinch of nutmeg or cumin. A nut of butter may be added at the last minute.

**Cream of oats soup**
Cook 6 tablespoons oats and 1 of wholemeal flour in a little butter or vegetable margarine till golden. Add a stick of celery and 2 litres (4 pints) of vegetable bouillon. Cook for an hour, strain, and add chopped chives and a table-spoonful of cream (optional) just before serving.

**Wholewheat soup**
Chop half an onion, half a leek and 2 or 3 sticks of celery. Cook in 10g (½ oz) butter until golden. Add 80g (3 oz) wholewheat (whole-grain or crushed) that has been soaked for 12 hours. Pour over 1 litre (1¾ pints) of vegetable bouillon, add a pinch of celery salt, and cook for a full hour. This may be put through blender before serving if wished.

**Minestrone**
1 tablespoon olive oil
1 tablespoon chopped onion
½ a leek, diced
¼ celery heart, chopped
1 carrot diced

2 or 3 cabbage leaves, cut in strips
1 or 2 potatoes, diced
A few leaves spinach or spinach-beet
Handful cooked haricot beans
2 ripe tomatoes
(Depending on the season, these vegetables may be varied
by the substitution of courgettes, green beans, peas, and so
on.) Sauté vegetables in the oil. Add a little thyme, basil,
oregano. Cook in 1 litre (1¾ pints) of water for about an
hour. A handful of cooked brown rice or wholemeal pasta
may be added shortly before the end of the cooking time.
Place 2 tablespoonfuls grated cheese in the tureen before
pouring in the soup. Leave in the oven for 15–20 minutes,
and just before serving add some chopped parsley.

## COOKED DISHES

### Soya balls
60g (2 oz) wholemeal flour
90g (3 oz) soya flour
200ml (7 oz) water
Mix the ingredients well, and beat until the paste forms
small bubbles. Leave for an hour. Form into small balls, and
drop them into boiling vegetable bouillon, removing them
when they rise to the surface. Serve with a little unsalted
butter, or cream (if tolerated).

### Spinach balls
60g (2 oz) wholemeal flour
20g (¾ oz) soya flour
200ml (7 oz) water
Large handful chopped spinach
Mix all the ingredients together into a smooth paste. Leave
for at least an hour. Then roll into balls and drop into
boiling water (or bouillon, if available). Remove when they

rise to the surface. Serve with tomato sauce, fried onions, or a little chopped parsley.

## Leaf spinach
1 kg (2 lbs) spinach, picked over and washed in salt water
1 small onion
1 clove garlic
Pinch of nutmeg
Chop the onion, and fry gently in a nut of butter with the garlic and nutmeg. Add the spinach and cook over a gentle heat. Before serving add 1 tablespoon melted butter and 1 tablespoon grated cheese.

## Petits pois à la française
½ onion
1 lettuce
500g (about 1 lb) fresh peas
Pinch of sugar
Fry the onion gently in a nut of butter or margarine. Add the lettuce, cut into quarters, the peas and sugar, with a large cup of vegetable bouillon. Cover and cook over a low heat for about half an hour. Then uncover and reduce the liquid. Season with chervil or parsley.

## Braised carrots
½ litre (1 pint) vegetable bouillon
750g (about 1½ lb) carrots, cut into rounds
1 tablespoon powdered sugar
Sprig of rosemary
Cook the carrots in bouillon for an hour, removing lid for last 10 minutes to reduce the liquid. Then add sugar and rosemary. When serving, add a nut of butter and some chopped parsley.

**Braised green beans**
1 onion (chopped)
1 clove of garlic
1kg (about 2 lb) french beans
1 tomato, seeded and chopped
Sprig of savory
Fry the onion and garlic lightly in a nut of butter or diet margarine. Add the beans, tomato and savory, cover and cook gently for about an hour. Before serving, sprinkle with parsley.

**Stuffed tomatoes**
Take 1 large or 2 small tomatoes per person. Slice off tops and remove seeds. Mix some cooked rice with chopped basil, chopped garlic and olive oil. Fill the tomatoes with this mixture, adding a pinch of sugar to each. Put the tops back on, and cook in a moderate oven for about half an hour.

**Stuffed potatoes**
1kg (about 2 lb) potatoes
200g (7 oz) low-fat soft cheese
½ litre (1 pt) milk
1 tablespoon cream (if tolerated)
Chopped chives or marjoram
Bake the potatoes in a moderate oven. When cooked, scoop out the insides and mix with the other ingredients (beating the cheese into the milk before adding it). Return mixture to potato shells and serve very hot.

## THE IMPORTANCE OF POTATOES

I should particularly like to point out the great value of potatoes. They are an important source of protein, especially where, as in some cultures, the staple food is restricted – to maize, for example. Recent nutritional experiments with five students carried out by Kofrany and Jekat gave some surprising results. They examined the protein of plant food (potatoes, wheat flour, maize, rice, seaweed, soya and kidney beans). The protein of potatoes was found to be equal to that of whole egg in terms of biological value and better than that of all other foods examined. The protein of the whole egg is supposed to have the highest biological value of all animal protein.

A mixture of 500g of potatoes plus one whole egg was found to be exceptional, resulting in the lowest daily protein requirement ever found by Kofrany and Jekat (24.2g per 70kg body weight).[1]

M. Mitrovic and N. Gladilin gave an account[2] of the important role of potatoes as food in those areas where pellagra (caused by deficiency of the vitamin niacin) is endemic. In the district of Mekomie in Yugoslavia, people live on maize almost exclusively. Maize is deficient in the essential amino-acids tryptophan and lysine. Potatoes are rich in lysine and tryptophan, a precursor for niacin.[3] Pellagra disappeared immediately when a daily supplement of 500g of potatoes per head had been supplied.


## DESSERTS

### Stewed rhubarb
1kg (about 2 lb) rhubarb
200g (7 oz) unrefined cane sugar

[1]E. Kofrany and F. Jekat, *Forscherbericht des Landes Nord-Rhein Westfahlen* No. 1582, p. 1 (1965).

[2]M. Mitrovic and N. Gladilin, 'Les diètes préventives et curatives de la pellagra endémique', Fourth International Congress on Nutrition, Paris, 1957.

[3]See also W. Schuphan, 'Control of plant proteins: the influence of genetics and ecology of food plants in proteins as human food', in *Proceedings* of the sixteenth Easter School in Agricultural Science, University of Nottingham, 1969, edited by Prof. R. A. Lawrie, Professor of Food Science, University of Nottingham School of Agriculture.

Wash and chop the rhubarb, and cook it with the sugar in very little water for 15–20 minutes, allowing the liquid to reduce. (Good for sluggish digestions)

**Fruit jelly**
300ml (10–11 oz) water, or grapejuice if available
60g (2½ oz) sugar
10g (½ oz) agar-agar (see the appendix on Types of Treatment)
100ml (3–4 oz) any fruit juice
Heat together the first three ingredients, stirring constantly, until the sugar and agar-agar are fully dissolved. Then add the fruit juice, still stirring. Pour into bowls or glasses and leave in refrigerator until set.

**Banana cream**
2 large bananas
1 tablespoon sugar
Few drops lemon juice
3 tablespoons cream or whipped cream
Purée the bananas in the blender. Then beat in the sugar and lemon juice. Finally, fold in the cream.

## FRUIT AND VEGETABLE JUICES

In cases of gastric or intestinal trouble, juices provide nourishment without giving the digestive system the strain of coping with solid food. All raw fruit and vegetables can be turned into juice. Wash them as described earlier. You will need a squeezer or an electric blender. And remember that all juices should be drunk as soon as they have been prepared.

Every fruit and vegetable has its own particular combination of mineral salts and vitamins. One should therefore make 'cocktails', not only to vary the flavour, but also to give as much nutritive value as possible. A few drops of lemon juice can always be added, and in some cases (ulcers or other gastro-intestinal ailments) it is a good idea to mix the juice with rice or barley water or linseed purée.

Here are some suggestions, but taste and experience will enable you to make your own combinations:
Equal parts of orange, mandarin and grapefruit juice.
One part persimmon to two parts of apple juice.

To either of these you can add – according to taste or dietary requirement – a few drops of lemon juice, honey, cream, or any vegetable milk (see below).
Equal parts of carrot, tomato and spinach juice.
Equal parts of tomato and carrot juice.
Equal parts of tomato and spinach juice.

You can always add interest to vegetable juices by including a little onion juice, sorrel, nettles (good for rheumatic complaints), chives, parsley, chervil, tarragon, or other herbs.

**Sauerkraut juice**
As a raw food, sauerkraut is digestible, and an excellent source of potassium. It is highly beneficial to the intestine. Squeeze 250g (about 8 oz) per person to make juice.

**Caution**: Potato juice must be made only from potatoes that have been washed and peeled and are thoroughly ripe. Do not use green or sprouting potatoes. This juice does not taste very pleasant, and should only be used for specific conditions, especially when there is gastro-intestinal inflammation.

## VEGETABLE MILKS

These may be bought from health-food shops, but they are not difficult to make. They can be drunk alone, or mixed with fruit juice. Either way, they are delicious.

## Almond milk
1½ tablespoons almonds
1 teaspoon honey
150ml (5–6 oz) water
Mix in blender and pass through a fine strainer. If fresh almonds are not available, substitute the same quantity of almond purée. This is rich in protein and very digestible.

## Pistachio milk
Prepare as almond milk. Very rich in fats and proteins.

## Sesame milk
1 tablespoon sesame purée
1 teaspoon lemon juice
1 teaspoon unrefined sugar
200ml (7 oz) water
Mix the first three ingredients, then add the water drop by drop, beating as with mayonnaise. This is delicious mixed in the blender with fresh bananas. Made with less water, it can be a pleasant substitute for fresh cream. Very rich in fatty acids.

# SEASONINGS

## Hot condiments
These are never allowed. All forms of pepper – white, black, cayenne, chilli – hot curry, and of course mustard, are irritants that can damage the intestinal wall and help to cause ulceration of the stomach.

## Salt
Except where a salt-free diet is indicated, sea-salt is allowed (since it contains other mineral salts as well as sodium). However, the body needs very little salt – half a gramme a day – and this can be provided by the salt present in our ordinary food in its natural state. Those who feel they

cannot do without the taste of additional salt should have no more than a maximum of 5g (a scant level teaspoon) a day.

Seasoning should enhance but never overpower the taste of food. But it is necessary, especially in diets where salt is forbidden (in heart or kidney complaints, overweight, and so on), to compensate for the lack of salt, pepper and strong spices. Furthermore, all the plants used for seasoning have their own medicinal value. The following are the ones most recommended in a Bircher-Benner diet:

**Anise**
Anise harmonises well with a number of vegetables and can be used in a great many dishes. Traditionally valued for its digestive and carminative properties.

**Basil**
Used to season salads, raw vegetables (especially tomatoes), soups, cream cheeses, courgettes, ratatouille. The dish in which it is best known is the Provençale *soupe au pistou*, in which pounded basil is added to a base of diced vegetables of all kinds, including three sorts of beans. Basil is considered a useful anti-spasmodic, with tonic and digestive properties, and has long been recommended for gastric spasms caused by nervous tension, and migraine of digestive or nervous origin.

**Bay-leaves**
These are used mainly in cooked dishes, especially as part of the traditional *bouquet garni*. They are thought to have a calming effect on all forms of spasm, coughs, stomach pains, vomiting, palpitations and insomnia.

**Borage**
Only use the small young leaves, which should be chopped

finely and added in small quantities to green salad or cucumber or potato salad. Borage flowers, which may be pink or blue, are edible, and make an attractive garnish for any dish of raw vegetables. Borage contains a large amount of potassium nitrate and is therefore used as a diuretic. Borage tea is used for colds, coughs, bronchitis, and catarrh.

## Celery
The leaves, stems and heart can all be used, cooked or raw, chopped up in soups or salads. A chemical analysis of celery would show essential oil, oleic acid, and valuable minerals, but no chemist could ever reconstitute these extracts as they are present naturally in the plant. Celery is considered tonic and anti-febrile, and stimulates the appetite.

## Chervil
Chop the leaves while fresh and add to green salads, other raw vegetable dishes, soups and sauces. Chervil goes with most things. Like parsley, it contains iron, but it can be taken in large amounts with no ill effect. It is used as a diuretic and stimulant.

## Chives
The mild onion flavour of chives harmonises well with all salads and raw vegetable dishes, but usually goes less well with cooked vegetables. Appetising and tasty.

## Cinnamon
The fragrance of cinnamon makes it especially delicious in stewed fruits. It can also be used sparingly in certain savoury cooked dishes, and adds piquancy to cream cheese. It contains starch, tannic acid and essential oil. Used to stimulate and arouse the muscular contractibility of the digestive system.

## Cloves
These are both aromatic and digestive. They can be used in small quantities in vegetable bouillons, and to flavour certain dishes. They contain essential oil, gum, resin and caryophyllin. A mild stimulant.

## Coriander
Coriander seeds are used a lot in Central Europe, to flavour wheat, pearl barley and most cereals. In France, Switzerland, Italy and England, they are used for pickling gherkins, among other things, and their use in cakes and breads dates back to the Romans. Considered digestive and carminative.

## Cumin
The roots, the young leaves and the seeds may all be used: they can be added to salads, vegetables, soups, potatoes. The seeds go particularly well with raw sauerkraut, soft cheese, and gherkins. Cumin has been used as an effective carminative, and to assist lactation.

## Dill
Young dill leaves may be chopped fine and added to cucumber or potato salad. Dill has the same stimulant, digestive and carminative properties as fresh anise, caraway, cumin, and fennel. Recommended for digestive problems and flatulence.

## Fennel
The young shoots and leaves should be chopped finely, and may be used in any salad, or to flavour raw juices. The seeds can be used to flavour bouillon, or when cooking vegetables or fish. Appetising and carminative; also diuretic.

**Garlic**
Cloves of garlic may be cooked with vegetables or used raw, chopped finely with parsley, to flavour salads. Garlic has remarkable medicinal properties: it is a natural disinfectant; it also stimulates the gastric juices and dissolves uric acid crystals. It is more digestible raw than cooked, but must be thoroughly chewed.

**Ginger**
Not everyone enjoys the strong taste of ginger. In powdered form it can be used to flavour fruit juices and stewed fruit. It speeds up the secretion of gastric juices and stimulates the digestion. It is also very useful for dyspepsia and colic. Chinese doctors claim that it stimulates the imagination and the brain.

**Horseradish**
Grated raw horseradish root can be added, in small quantities, to salad dressing and other sauces. It has valuable stimulant, diuretic and antiseptic properties.

**Lemon balm (Melissa)**
The young leaves, cut or chopped like parsley, are delicious in salads and harmonise well with other herbs. Courgettes cooked with lemon balm make an unusual and mouthwatering dish. Lemon balm is well known as a digestive (melissa water). It is also used as a sudorific and antispasmodic.

**Marjoram (or Oregano)**
Adds flavour to salads, raw vegetables, herb and vegetable soups. Marjoram contains camphor and is recommended for a sluggish stomach, gastric acidity, and for catarrh and asthma. Also an anti-spasmodic.

## Mint

There are several types of mint, both wild and cultivated, but most people will be using the common garden mint. The young leaves, finely chopped, may be used with other herbs in any salad, and give a delicious flavour to tomato-based dishes, such as ratatouille and tomato sauce. Mint is also one of the most digestive of all plants, as well as having anti-spasmodic and tonic properties.

## Nettles

These add a pleasant flavour to vegetable juices, spinach and soups. The juice of the common nettle has been used as a vaso-constrictor and to stop diarrhoea in acute and chronic enteritis. It is also said to stimulate the reproductive functions. Pick only young leaves that are fresh and tender.

## Onions

Finely chopped onion is used to flavour all salads and is the basis of many other dishes. The bulb contains salts, oxydases and amylases with a marked diuretic action, but these disappear when heated. Onions should therefore preferably be eaten raw. Since they contain little starch, they are a useful food for varying the menu of diabetics.

## Parsley

Parsley could be described as a miniature mineral salt processing factory. It gives a mild stimulus to the brain, and contains salts beneficial to anyone suffering from physical fatigue. 10g (½ oz) of parsley eaten every day prevents dark rings under the eyes. *Caution*: in excessive amounts, parsley can produce dizziness and symptoms of intoxication.

**Rosemary**
Adds flavour to rice, potatoes, ratatouille and all Provencal dishes. Small quantities of powdered rosemary may be added to vegetable juices. Its essential oil is a stomach stimulant, valuable in cases of sluggish digestion.

**Sage**
Sage goes particularly well with some vegetables, such as haricot beans, to which it gives a delicious flavour. It is considered digestive and carminative, and is recommended to anyone who is prone to dizziness.

**Salad burnet**
This is used in salads, mixtures of aromatic herbs, soups and vegetables, and goes very well with parsley and celery. Burnet is used as an astringent in cases of diarrhoea, dysentery and enteritis. It stimulates the appetite and helps digestion.

**Savory**
Savory makes a delicious seasoning for beans, tomatoes and ratatouille, and is very good in salads, providing the central stem is removed and only the young shoots used. They should be chopped very finely. Savory has the same medicinal uses as thyme, and is said to stimulate the reproductive functions.

**Shallots**
Cooked or raw, they give an excellent flavour to salads or cooked dishes. But they should be used more sparingly than onions because, though they have similar diuretic value, they also cause flatulence.

**Tarragon**
Tarragon does not go with all vegetables, for its unique

flavour can clash with others. It is excellent with tomatoes, lettuce, potatoes (especially potato salad), and cucumbers. Particularly recommended to anyone suffering from loss of appetite, gastritis or rheumatic complaints.

## Thyme

The flowers are delicious in green salads and all raw vegetable salads. Thyme is part of the bouquet garni used in cooking; it is also used in pickling gherkins, onions, etc. Assists the digestion; an excellent disinfectant, and a good pick-me-up, especially for children. Has a similar diuretic effect to rosemary.

# INFUSIONS

The fact that herbal infusions are so often used in diets should not mislead anyone into thinking that they are purely medicinal; indeed, they are very often delicious as well. Unless otherwise stated, use approximately 1 teaspoonful of dried herbs per cup.

## Soothing teas

*Camomile:* Pour boiling water on to camomile flowers and leave to infuse for a few minutes. *Caution:* too concentrated an infusion can cause vomiting.
*Lemon verbena:* Prepare as camomile tea.
*Lemon-peel tea:* Make sure that you use only untreated lemons. Wash a lemon and pare off the zest. This is then cooked gently in ½ litre (1 pint) of water for 5 minutes. Leave to stand for 10 minutes, then strain.

## Sleep-inducing teas

*Lemon-balm tea:* Pour boiling water on to the leaves. Allow to infuse for 5 minutes, then sweeten with honey and drink before going to bed.

*Lime-flower tea:* Prepare as lemon-balm tea.
*Orange-flower tea:* Put the flowers in water (2 or 3 flowers per cup) and boil for 2–3 minutes.

## Digestive teas
*Wormwood tea:* Pour boiling water over the wormwood and infuse for 5 minutes. Can be sipped throughout the day.
*Peppermint tea:* Prepare as wormwood tea.
Camomile and lime-flower tea also assist digestion.

## Diuretic teas
*Golden-rod tea:* Boil 2 tablespoonfuls of leaves in ½ litre (1 pint) water for 1 minute, then leave to infuse for 10 minutes. Drink 2–3 cups a day.
*Rose-hip:* 2–3 tablespoonfuls to ½ litre (1 pint) water. Steep for 12 hours, simmer in the same water for half an hour, then strain.
*Horse-tail:* Prepare as golden-rod tea.

## To prevent flatulence
A tea made of equal parts of cumin, fennel and anise seeds. Add to water that has just boiled, and infuse for 20 minutes. A cup may be drunk after every meal.

## Bitter tea
Equal parts of wormwood, centaury and avens (also called colewort or herb bennet). Add to boiling water and infuse for 5 minutes. Two or three tablespoonfuls before meals will relieve biliousness.

## Teas for stomach upsets
*Sage:* A few leaves to a breakfast-cup of boiling water. Leave to infuse for 5 minutes. Very good for the gall bladder.

*Thyme:* Two or three small sprigs of thyme to a breakfast-cup of water. Boil for 1 minute and infuse for 5 minutes. Drink after meals.
*Rosemary:* As thyme tea.

**A rejuvenating tea**
**(excellent for women at the menopause)**
Equal quantities of applemint and witch-hazel. Pour boiling water on to the herbs and leave to infuse for 5 minutes.

# 10. Illnesses and their Treatments

The 'strict diets' described must never be undertaken without medical authority and supervision, and some must only be followed in a clinic.[1]

On the other hand, there can be no danger in undertaking the 'overhaul' treatment (see Detoxication, p. 127). It is advisable to spend a week on a Bircher-Benner diet at every change of season, concentrating on the seasonal fruits and vegetables. Indeed, if you either cannot or do not want to adopt this new way of life permanently, it is still very beneficial to change to it for a week of every month.

Whichever course you decide upon, it is vital to cut down on salt, and to cut out altogether all hot spices, stimulants, alcohol, tobacco, chocolate, confectionery and all animal fats other than very small quantities of butter and cream as specified. When on a strict diet even decaffeinated coffee is not allowed, and herb teas are restricted. Water may be drunk freely except where the aim is to lose weight, when consumption of fluids must be cut down.

## ACNE

The term 'acne' is used of all skin problems caused by the abnormal activity of the sebaceous glands. Adolescents are made miserable by these 'spots', which are unsightly and can leave scars.

The sebaceous glands are most active on the forehead, cheeks, chest, and back. They secrete sebum, a greasy substance that lubricates the skin. When they secrete too much of it (seborrhea) the skin becomes shiny. It used to be

[1] Dr Bircher-Benner's clinic still exists: Privat-Klinic Dr Bircher-Benner, Keltenstrasse 48, 8044 Zurich.

thought that seborrhea was related solely to these glands, but it is now realised that in adolescence, with the onset of puberty (in girls it occurs at the end of the menstrual cycle), a sudden increase of the male hormone stimulates the production of sebum – which in turn clogs up the skin and causes blackheads. If bacteria (usually staphylococcal) enter the swollen gland-openings the minor local infection called acne is produced.

Most people think acne is more of a cosmetic problem than an illness. But this is quite wrong. It is important that the root cause of acne is discovered and removed. At a time when others were ready to blame it solely on sexual deprivation, Bircher-Benner came to realise that acne has psychological causes. But a psychosomatic illness can take hold only where the ground is prepared, and in this case a diet rich in fats and lacking in vitamins (especially vitamin $B_1$), poor hygiene, alcohol and too many stimulants fertilise the soil wonderfully.

If you suffer from acne, adopt the following programme the moment the first spots appear:

1 Give up alcohol and all stimulants (tea, coffee, and so on).

2 Stop using face creams, and give up ordinary soap. Instead use an acid pH soap.

3 Twice a day – on getting up and going to bed – apply very hot and very cold water friction alternately to stimulate circulation.

4 Expose your skin to the sun, or a sun-lamp. But be careful – this should be done gradually, starting with a quarter of an hour, and never exceeding an hour. A sun-lamp should only be used under supervision, since nothing is more dangerous for the skin than strong ultra-violet rays.

5 Diet as follows, selecting foods rich in vitamins A, $B_1$, $B_2$ and $B_6$ (see Vitamin Table).

(i)  *Take a vegetable laxative, and then fast on fluids only for two days:*
    *Morning:* 200g (7 oz) fresh fruit juice
               150g (5 oz) almond milk
               1 cup of rose-hip tea
    *Midday:* 200g (7 oz) fresh fruit juice
               150g (5 oz) vegetable juice
               150g (5 oz) soya milk
    *Evening:* As morning

(ii)  *For one week:*
    *Morning:* 250g (9 oz) muesli with almond purée, using apples or whatever fruit is in season and any nuts except peanuts.
               When mixing the muesli, add a spoonful of flaked yeast, rich in vitamin B.
    *Midday:* Fresh fruit and almonds – as much as you like
               Raw vegetables and germinated cereals
    *Evening:* As morning, with the addition of dried fruit, such as raisins or figs

(iii)  *For one month:*
    *Morning:* Muesli with almond purée
               Fruit according to season
               Wholemeal bread with 10g (½ oz) butter or vegetable margarine
               Herb tea
    *Midday:* Fresh fruit
               Raw vegetables
               Cooked cereals or vegetables or soup
               Dessert
               Rose-hip tea
    *Evening:* As morning, or Fruit

> Soup
> Wholemeal bread
> Stewed fruit
> Herb tea

(iv)  *Until completely better:*
  *Morning:* Muesli
  Fruit
  Wholemeal bread with butter or vege-
  table margarine
  Herb tea
  *Midday:* Fruit
  Raw vegetables
  Two dishes of cooked vegetables and
  cereals
  Dessert
  *Evening:* Muesli or fruit salad with yoghourt
  Wholemeal bread with butter or vege-
  table margarine
  Soft low-fat cheese

Always remember that constipation can cause an attack of acne. If this diet does not get rid of it, mild enemas may be used until normal action returns (see appendix on Types of Treatment).

## AGEING

Some people never let themselves get old – why should you? Old age is a psychosomatic illness. As long as you feel young, nothing is going to get you down, physically or mentally. People talk of 'growing old gracefully', and of how 'every age has its pleasures' – but these are confessions of defeat. The human machine is built to last eighty or ninety years, and there is no reason for it to stop working well. Like any other machine, however, it does need a certain amount of care and maintenance.

If you want to stay young, never forget that:

Obesity is ageing: it is physically tiring and mentally depressing, and it leads to illness.

Poor circulation causes serious degenerative illnesses, such as phlebitis and arteriosclerosis.

The digestive organs that filter and transform our food – mouth, stomach, intestines, liver, kidneys – must not be overburdened with too much 'waste material' or food that cannot be put to good use in the body.

The heart must not be overworked.

Recent scientific discoveries, often confirming what our ancestors believed empirically, have made it possible to withstand wear and tear more effectively. For instance, we now understand the value of wheatgerm: hence the importance of eating wholemeal bread rather than white.

Another example, and one which has long been taboo, is sexuality. We now know that the sex glands do more than ensure reproduction. They vitalise the body. You must not let them become idle, on the grounds that 'I'm too old for that sort of thing'. There is no such thing as being too old if you remain young in mind. And if those glands show signs of flagging, you must get them working again, just as you would any other organ. Nature has made everything we need available to us – plants contain the same sexual substances as we do. When bulls get old, breeders have always added oats to their food. In the past, when a woman came to the village wise woman because she was unable to conceive, she would be given nettle seeds. Modern biochemical research has discovered the wise woman's secret: there are 14,000 units of oestrogen in every kilogramme of nettles, and, as we know, oestrogens are the hormones that enable women to ovulate. Oat-, wheat- and rice-germ all contain large amounts of sexual substances, as do all tubers, celery and dandelions, and such aromatic herbs as sage, mint, savory and parsley.

A research chemist, Dr Loewe, has recently demonstrated the presence of male hormones in certain catkins. Paradoxically, plants are more 'highly-sexed' than people, so from middle age we should all try to have a diet rich in sex hormones (present in far larger quantities in vegetables than in meat products), while women should take vitamin A and men vitamin E (see Vitamin Table). The detoxication diet given later (p. 127) makes a good basis, and one can, in addition, adopt a menu such as the following on one or two days each month:

|  |  |
|---|---|
| *Morning:* | Muesli |
|  | Raw fruit |
|  | Mint tea |
| *Midday:* | Raw fruit |
|  | Celery salad, with corn oil, lemon juice and parsley |
|  | Cream of oatmeal soup (p. 94) |
|  | Wholemeal bread |
|  | Leaf spinach (p. 96) |
| *Evening:* | Muesli or fruit |
|  | Artichoke vinaigrette (with corn oil) |
|  | Low-fat soft cheese |

## ARTERIOSCLEROSIS

Arterial disease is *the* illness of our time. Arteriosclerosis is a thickening and hardening of the walls of the arteries, by deposits of fat and cholesterol – which then become hard, weakening the arteries so that they lose their elasticity, and sometimes become completely blocked. The inadequate flow of blood that results has various ill effects: heart failure, angina, coronary thrombosis, lesions of the arteries, inflammation of the kidneys.

Though the illnesses may not appear until late in life,

the damage takes place much earlier, often in a person's twenties. Predisposing factors of risk are a sedentary life, heavy smoking, high blood pressure, prolonged periods of mental or emotional stress, diabetes, obesity, thyroid deficiency, and bad eating habits, especially an excess of animal protein.

As a young doctor, Max Bircher-Benner pinpointed diet as the cause of arteriosclerosis – he saw proof of it daily in his consulting-room. Farmers, whose diet was frugal but healthy, never suffered from it, whereas prosperous tradesmen and city-dwellers, fond of their beer and their lavish dinners, very often did.

Some twenty years ago, a young doctor did an autopsy on an Eskimo in Greenland, a man of twenty-four: to his astonishment, he found the young man had died of arteriosclerosis. This contradicted all his previous medical experience, but he then discovered that Greenlanders, at whatever age they died, almost always died of the same thing. The explanation was simple: they ate almost no green vegetables or fruit, and had too much meat (often uncooked) and fats.

This is an illness to be prevented rather than cured – or at least to be prevented from getting worse. This is what you must do:

1 Watch your weight, your cholesterol level and your blood pressure. If any of these are high there is danger.

2 Keep away from over-rich food, spirits and stimulants, and avoid laxatives and tranquillisers.

3 If you find yourself getting unusually tense, overtired, or out of breath, consult your doctor and put yourself on a diet. (The Bircher-Benner diet will be found in the section on High Cholesterol Level, p. 138.)

Remember, if you suffer from arteriosclerosis, cellulose and vitamin E are both very important. Both are present in large quantities in whole wheat, soya beans, wheatgerm and wheatgerm oil, walnuts, and linseed and sunflower oils.


## ARTHRITIS

The Royal Free Hospital in London was the first to recognise Dr Bircher-Benner's unequalled authority in the treatment of rheumatism, and the spectacular results he achieved.

In 1936 the hospital had one woman patient who was almost totally paralysed by arthritis. Every possible treatment was tried, if only to relieve her pain, but all failed. One of the doctors suggested sending her to Zurich as a last hope. The woman spent several months at the Bircher-Benner clinic. She had arrived bedridden, and she went home completely cured. The English doctors were cautious: to prove that hers had not been an isolated case, or merely a coincidence, they decided to try the Bircher-Benner treatment in their own hospital on twelve arthritics believed to be incurable. They chronicled their progress on film.

That film provided overwhelming evidence. It showed the twelve patients at the beginning, all immobile in their beds and totally dependent on their nurses. Then, as the days passed, these human statues began to come to life: the foot of one would move; the head, the fingers, of others. The look of joy on their faces told its own story. Seven of them walked away from the hospital carrying their own suitcases; three others showed a marked improvement – no more pain, no more pain-killers, and hope where there had been none before. Only two were not helped.

There is nothing magic about the Bircher-Benner cure, and it is not hard to follow. Arthritis is an inflammation of the joints due to degeneration of the connective tissue. That tissue is somewhat like a fine layer of spongy rubber around the bones and cavities of the joints, and it degenerates if the normal intestinal flora disappear. People with chronic constipation are therefore almost always potential, if not actual, arthritis sufferers. Healthy intestinal flora can be restored by a diet of raw fruit and vegetables because of the enzymes they contain. Such a diet also assists the arthritic by generally ridding the system of poisons, and especially those affecting the soft connective tissue.

Chronic rheumatoid arthritis is not a dangerous illness in the sense that no one dies from it – but it can result in a living death that barely seems preferable. The Royal Free's experiments showed that, with the Bircher-Benner treatment, there is considerable hope of recovery. But it is important to have the willpower and patience to observe the rules strictly.

## 1 Eliminating all sources of infection
At the start of an arthritic attack, there is very often some source of infection to be found – the two most common being teeth and tonsils. In any form of neuralgia, it is vital to have a dental check-up: a decayed tooth you are not even aware of can do a lot of damage.

## 2 Therapeutic diet
The patient must eat nothing but raw food for at least 3–4 weeks, and no animal fat or protein. Permitted foods are as follows:

Fresh fruit juice: any

Fresh vegetable juice: any

Raw fruit: any, including walnuts and almonds

Raw vegetables: any, including sauerkraut and potatoes, and plenty of cabbage and onions

Aromatic herbs: parsley, chervil, chives, garlic, thyme, basil, savory, sage, rosemary, tarragon

Dressings: lemon juice and small quantities of vegetable oil

Cereals: raw, and in muesli

When you feel there has been real improvement, you may add:

Fresh vegetable bouillon

Cooked vegetables, including potatoes in their jackets

Fats: a maximum of 20g (¾ oz) butter per day

Cheese: small quantities of soft white or cottage cheese

Wholemeal bread: 2–3 slices per day

*Absolutely no* meat, fish, shellfish, tinned food, milk products or cheese other than those mentioned, eggs, salt, spices, coffee, alcohol, or tobacco. Although the diet may take months to bring about a cure, or even a marked improvement, there is almost always considerable improvement in the end.

**3  External treatment** (see Appendix for descriptions of the various Types of Treatment)

(i) *Physiotherapy*

In acute arthritic attacks (fever, swollen joints, pain, and possibly even heart pains):

Complete bed rest; Priessnitz packs; the application of cabbage leaves to the affected joints;[1] cold compresses of water and clay; sun lamp treatment; relaxation.

In chronic arthritis (sensitivity to cold, stiffness, joints becoming misshapen and immobile):

Hot baths: these can be varied, using herbs, clay, mud, sulphur, horse-chestnut essence

Baths of hot sand for the hands

Sunbathing; sun-lamp

(ii) *Stimulating hydrotherapy*

Alternating showers, Kneipp douches; saunas are also helpful.

---

[1] Raw cabbage, pounded with pestle and mortar, should be applied directly to the skin, covered with a blanket, and left for about 20 minutes.

(iii) *Maintenance Physiotherapy*
As you start to feel better, you must re-educate your body with the help of a trained physiotherapist. You should also observe the following rules:
Lead a calm and regular life.
Take enough exercise to keep you fit, but not overtire you, such as walking, gymnastics, and games that are not too strenuous.
Daily 'air bathing', and sunbathing whenever possible.
Daily 'alternating showers'.
Make sure you get eight hours' sleep a night.

## COLITIS

Colitis sufferers tend to be people in a hurry or under stress, or those who eat a lot of starchy food. Colitis may start by being no more than an inflammation of the colon, but it can turn into a real problem if it becomes chronic. The symptoms are irregular sharp pains over a part of the stomach, great distension after meals and flatulence: sufferers also complain of migraines, of burning ears and faces, of difficulty in breathing, palpitations, sleepiness, heaviness in the legs and bad temper. There may also be diarrhoea or constipation. All these symptoms are intensified by emotion, worry, and any change of diet or lifestyle. Psychological factors are therefore clearly involved, and we must seek to get at the 'root of the illness'. The doctor may find a specific physical cause: intestinal parasites, amoebic dysentery, reliance on laxatives. But in many cases the main cause of the trouble is faulty eating, so the Bircher-Benner cure can have a marked effect.

Acute attacks of colitis, however dramatic and agonising, are seldom dangerous. The worst feature of the illness is that it can become chronic and dominate a person's life. In the Bircher-Benner cure there are six main points to remember:

1 Anyone with gastric or intestinal problems should eat slowly, chewing each mouthful thoroughly, and should lie down for ten minutes before every meal and for half an hour afterwards.

2 Cut out all alcohol, coffee, chocolate, sweets and cakes, and tobacco.

3 Raw fruit and vegetables should always be eaten before any other food, though in acute attacks they must be purée'd.

4 Go for walks: walking is a natural massage which stimulates the digestive organs.

5 Learn to relax and avoid stress. It is particularly important to be calm and relaxed during meals.

6 If there is constipation, it must be dealt with properly, and not ignored.

If the attack is very painful, relief can be had from hayflower baths (see appendix) and from hot packs – which should be replaced with cold Priessnitz packs when the pain is reduced.

The following diet is recommended in cases of colitis:

**1  For one week:**

Fruit juices: grapefruit, mandarin, grape, apple, peach, plum, melon.

Vegetable juices: carrot, beetroot, lettuce, celery, fennel, black radish, spinach. Mix 2 parts of juice with 1 of linseed, or wholewheat purée, rice or barley water. You may add cream, pectin or agar-agar (see appendix). 600–800g (20–30 oz) to be drunk over the course of a day. Also take 100g (3–4 oz) raw cabbage juice and 50g (2 oz) potato juice.

Cereal purée: linseed, wholewheat – 2–5 cups per day.

Infusions: as preferred – but if flatulence is a problem the best are blackberry-leaf or strawberry-leaf: 1 litre to be drunk during the course of a day, unsweetened, with 5–10 drops of lemon juice per cup.

For constipation, have a camomile enema (1 litre) every other day.

*Caution:* citrus fruit should only be eaten if there are no contra-indications; spinach juice may not be tolerated at all, but if it is, only 1 tablespoonful per day, mixed with carrot juice, should be drunk.

**2 For the next few weeks, until there is real improvement:**

Fresh fruit: grated finely or mashed (apples, pears, peaches, melons, bananas). Unlike traditional diets, very little or no cooked fruit.

Fresh vegetables: all raw vegetables, except cabbage, which should be taken only in the form of juice. Purée them in a blender or mince finely. Dress lightly with pure oil, lemon juice, purée of almonds. Eat immediately.

Cooked vegetables: blend or pass through a sieve; add a nut of (uncooked) butter.

Dairy products: milk alone or in mixed dishes (such as muesli), yoghourt, buttermilk, low-fat cheese (soft cheese can be mixed with a spoonful of yeast extract). If tolerated, a small amount of cream may be taken to make your food more interesting.

Vegetable milks: soya, almond and sesame.

Cereals: whole wheat, brown rice, whole barley, whole oats; eaten as porridge, or ground and raw, or in wholemeal bread or crispbread.

Fats: cold-pressed vegetable oils only (pure olive oil, sunflower oil, cereal-germ oils); small quantities of butter (uncooked and *never* mixed with oil).

Sweetening: only honey and unrefined brown sugar.

Eggs: if tolerated – one egg-yolk once or twice a week, beaten into vegetable juice or soup.

Meat: if you must have meat, eat only 150g (5–6 oz) of lean meat, grilled, no more than once or twice a week.

Drinks: fresh fruit juices, herb teas, non-sparkling mineral waters.

*Absolutely no* fried foods, cooked fats, refined flour or sugar, or stimulants.

**3  For 2–3 months you should keep to the following diet:**
Fresh fruit: any.

Raw vegetables: any, but it is wiser to avoid onions, spring onions, shallots and chives.

Cooked vegetables: avoid peas, potatoes and tomatoes. Eat no more than one or two different vegetables at one meal. They should preferably be steamed, without any sauce or thickening – though a little cornflour may occasionally be used. *Never* eat cooked cabbage, only raw cabbage or sauerkraut.

Dairy products: milk alone or in prepared dishes (e.g. muesli), yoghourt, buttermilk, low-fat soft cheese.

Vegetable milks: soya, almond.

Cereals: wholemeal bread, pumpernickel bread, crispbread. Corn, barley, oats, rice (all whole) in soup or porridge. A little pasta can be eaten, but only once a week.

Fats: olive and sunflower oil; unsalted butter; cream.

Sweetening: only unrefined brown sugar and pure honey.

Eggs: in any form other than fried, but no more than 2 per week.

Meat: only lean, grilled, and no more often than twice a week.

Drinks, fresh fruit juices, herb teas, and non-sparkling mineral waters.

*Absolutely no* roast meats, sauces, confectionary, stimulants.

As a *general rule,* it is preferable to have several small

meals in the day. Large amounts of food eaten at a time – even nutritionally excellent food – are harmful. It is easier to digest smaller quantities. It is also wise to avoid having too many different dishes, so that you are not tempted to eat more.

## CONSTIPATION

Constipation is often believed (wrongly) to be one of life's minor trials, and is philosophically accepted as something one just has to put up with. Chronic constipation, because it poisons the system, can lead to serious problems, to say nothing of such harmless but unpleasant symptoms as pimples, blotchy skin, bad breath, and headaches. An intestine that is emptied daily is the prime guarantee of good health. Many doctors consider constipation a female ailment, though they cannot say precisely why. Traditional medicine is all too often helpless to deal with it.

Whether it originates from persistent chronic colitis or a sluggishness encouraged by the kind of busy life which often makes it impossible to respond at once to the urge to defecate, constipation must be overcome. One of the most frequent causes is reliance on laxatives: these make the intestine irremediably lazy by artificially and rapidly causing the peristaltic movements that should occur spontaneously. They irritate and, be they vegetable or mineral, their effect is much too drastic and causes the loss of mineral salts (especially potassium). Finally, and most serious of all, they prepare a favourable ground for cancer by keeping the intestinal wall in a permanent state of irritation.

The Bircher-Benner treatment can have the most spectacular effect on constipation. It disappears totally in a few weeks. But it is vital not to abandon the programme for even a day, and absolutely no laxative medicines must be taken.

1 So long as the treatment continues, eat no food other than the following:

Fresh fruit: whatever is in season, plus stewed rhubarb (see p. 98)

Dried fruit: figs, prunes, pears

Fresh vegetables: concentrate on green, raw vegetables. Have three kinds of salad at midday, with plenty of green leaves. Also raw sauerkraut and the water from it.

Cereals: germinated wheat, diet foods with a bran base, muesli, wholewheat porridge, linseed purée (this last is especially recommended for constipation)

Fats: any vegetable oil

Dairy products: yoghourt, buttermilk, sour milk

Drinks: herb tea sweetened with honey, apple juice

2 Exercise and hydrotherapy are important. Go for walks. Your abdomen should be treated with alternating douches and cold water friction using a clockwise motion (see appendix on Types of Treatment).

3 Do not take any laxative medicines. Before going to bed at night you may take 1 or 2 spoonfuls of psyllium seed or linseed infusion (see appendix) or a cup of boldo-leaf tea. Try all three, and stick to the one that suits you best. At the end of a week or so, you should find you need it only every other day, then every three days. Half-way through the treatment, you should find that you no longer need anything.

Once these few weeks are over, depending on results, you can consolidate your cure by carrying on with the same diet for another month, but adding to it: wholemeal bread, butter, steamed vegetables, potatoes, whole-grain cereals.

To make sure there is no recurrence, it is advisable to cut out permanently: white bread and flour, white sugar and rice, chocolate, coffee, alcohol and all 'heating' food, such as meat, especially game and rich sauces.

At the first sign of a recurrence, return to the treatment for a week. The more you revert to your old eating habits, the more likely such unpleasant recurrences will be. You can only get rid of the problem permanently by sticking as closely as possible to the Bircher-Benner diet system.

## DETOXICATION

To cleanse your system, try this 8-day cure:
    3 days on raw fruit and vegetables only
    2 days' mixed diet
    1 day's transition diet
    2 days' regular Bircher-Benner diet

1 *Three days of raw fruit and vegetables:*
  *Morning:*  Muesli with germinated wheat
                Fresh fruit as available (only apple if your liver is very damaged)
                Rose-hip tea
  *Midday:*  First day:    Raw fruit
                         Celery, tomatoes, lettuce
          Second day:  Fresh fruit
                         Beetroot, cucumber, lettuce
          Third day:   Fresh fruit or fruit juice
                         Carrots, celeriac, watercress
  *Evening:*  As morning

2 *Two days' mixed diet: the same as above, but add*
  *Morning:*  1 slice of wholewheat or pumpernickel bread
                5g (¼ oz) butter
  *Midday:*  Vegetable bouillon, potatoes, haricot beans
  *Evening:*  As morning

3 *One day's transition diet*
  *Morning:* Fruit
            Muesli
            2 slices of wholemeal bread with about 15g
            (½ oz) butter
            Yoghourt
            Rose-hip tea
  *Midday:* Fruit
            Raw vegetables: cauliflower, spinach, lettuce
            Soup (any kind)
  *Evening:* As morning, but honey or jam may be added

4 *Two days' normal Bircher-Benner diet*
  *Morning:* As transition day
  *Midday:* First day:     Fruit
                           Dressed raw vegetables: carrots,
                           beetroot, lettuce
                           Wholewheat soup (see p. 94)
                           Spinach
                           Stuffed potatoes (see p. 97).
            Second day:    Fruit
                           Salad of raw vegetables: celery,
                           watercress, lettuce
                           Cooked vegetables: courgettes,
                           mashed potatoes
                           Fruit jelly (see p. 99).
  *Evening:* First day:    As morning, but with addition
                           of low-fat soft cheese
            Second day:    Muesli
                           Minestrone
                           Wholemeal bread with butter
    Don't hesitate to repeat this detoxication cure as often as
you feel the need of it. As well as being worth doing in

itself, it also develops your taste for the Bircher-Benner diet system, and helps you to form new eating habits.

## ENTERITIS

Serious enteritis, with ulceration and the passing of blood or mucus, must of course be treated by a doctor. But slight diarrhoea – due to eating the wrong food, taking too many laxatives, or travelling – should not be neglected, since it may become chronic. Here is a safe and effective treatment:

1  A camomile enema every two days, to cleanse the intestine of all impurities (see appendix on Types of Treatment).

2  Hot packs or compresses after meals, and cold ones at night when the body is warm in bed.

3  Rest, in bed if possible.

4  A soothing infusion, such as camomile, will ease discomfort.

5  Breathing exercises will assist relaxation (tension intensifies pain).

6  Have three meals a day, at regular times, until you are fully recovered. They should consist of:

Fresh fruit and vegetable juices

Vegetable bouillon

Dairy products: 2 or 3 yoghourts a day (more if possible); 150g (5–6 oz) whey or fresh buttermilk.

Vegetable milks: almond or sesame (see p. 101), 150g (5–6 oz) per day.

Drinks: herb tea or water.

This rigid diet can gradually be extended to include muesli, then raw vegetables, and finally cooked vegetables and brown rice, thus bringing you back by easy stages to normal eating.

## FATIGUE

This does not mean the kind of healthy tiredness that comes at the end of a day's work, when a good night's sleep is all that's needed to restore your energy.

More and more people nowadays complain of a chronic sense of fatigue: they wake feeling tired and, though they can overcome it for a few hours, it gradually returns as the day goes on. It may be the symptom of a latent illness – anaemia, diabetes, tuberculosis, an intestinal parasite, underactive thyroid, adrenal deficiency, some concealed infection. It is vital to have a thorough medical check so that the cause can be treated rather than the symptom. To mask the effects of fatigue by administering stimulant drugs, or keeping yourself going with coffee or alcohol, is foolish in the extreme. Fatigue, like fever and pain, is a warning sign that requires attention.

But the fatigue people feel today is often due to the stress of modern life and the insomnia that is the price they pay for driving themselves on. Another and even more potent cause, because they are not aware of it, is an unbalanced diet, often gulped down at high speed. Fatigue of this kind yields rapidly to the Bircher-Benner treatment, and since it is easy to follow, even at home, it works.

1 First of all, examine your psychological and emotional state. Fatigue is often at least partly psychosomatic. A repressed worry, like an abscess that refuses to come to a head, can infect the entire body. It is better to discover what the trouble is and confront the problem openly. Dr Bircher-Benner used to say to people, 'Your fatigue is your responsibility. It's up to you to find the cause.'

2 Try to do a little less for a while. It is better to work and play less for a few weeks than to get to a point where you have to give up altogether.

3 Follow a diet that will both cleanse your system and

restore your own life force, the dynamism you are now lacking.

While on the diet, it is desirable to stay in bed – at least for the first forty-eight hours. It is a good idea, therefore, to start your cure on a Saturday or Sunday. We don't expect to have to work over the weekend, but when our bodies demand a weekend's rest too, we pay no attention. In fact, they often work harder then, because of the large meals we tend to have.

(i) *The first day*
    *Morning:* 200g (7 oz) fresh fruit juice
    *Midday:* 200g (7 oz) fresh vegetable juice with a squeeze of lemon
    *Evening:* 200g (7 oz) orange juice
    Two cups of golden-rod tea during the day

(ii) *The second day*
    *Morning:* Muesli with apple and yoghourt
    200g (7 oz) fresh fruit juice
    *Midday:* One raw vegetable
    200g (7 oz) fresh vegetable juice with a squeeze of lemon
    *Evening:* If you are hungry, a helping of muesli in addition to your
    200g (7 oz) fruit juice

(iii) *For one week*
    *Morning:* 200g (7 oz) fresh fruit juice
    1 yoghourt or muesli or helping of raw cereal with fruit
    *Midday:* Fruit, raw vegetables
    Cooked vegetables or cereals
    *Evening:* Fresh fruit, muesli
    1 slice wholemeal bread

Low-fat soft cheese
Rose-hip tea may be drunk with meals

(iv)  *For at least one month*
 *Morning:* Raw fruit
    Muesli
 *Midday:* Raw fruit
    Salad of raw vegetables
    2 dishes of cooked vegetables, or soup
    and 1 dish of cooked vegetables
    Wholemeal bread
    Dessert
 *Evening:* Raw fruit
    Muesli
    Wholemeal bread and low-fat or cottage cheese.
 Rose-hip tea may be drunk with meals.
*Note:* Germinated wheat and raw cereals are very energising, so they are important in combating fatigue.

4  As long as the treatment continues, you should observe the following daily routine.

(i) If possible have a half-hour's walk every morning – you might walk to work, but leave in good time to walk, not run! At the weekend try to have long, unhurried walks in the country.

(ii) Have alternate hot and cold showers morning and evening (see appendix on Types of Treatment).

(iii) Rest for half an hour after lunch, in the sun if possible.

(iv) Walk for half an hour after dinner.

(v) Go to bed at nine o'clock. If you suffer from insomnia, have a large cup of lime-flower tea.

## GASTRITIS

Like colitis, gastritis can begin with mild symptoms, then become serious or persistent. In this case it is the mucous membrane of the stomach that is inflamed. The symptoms are acidity or heartburn, flatulence and sometimes diarrhoea. The cause may be a hangover, food that has been cooked too long, or food that is slightly off – eggs or shellfish, perhaps. It is important to discover the cause rather than merely treating the symptoms, otherwise you will either be permanently on 'indigestion tablets' or find that you dare not eat any but the most bland foods.

Chronic gastritis can be a symptom of serious illness, and you must consult your doctor about it. But, where the main cause of gastritis is bad eating habits, the Bircher-Benner treatment brings rapid relief.

1 The first two or three days:

Soothing infusions – camomile, linseed, rose-hip, marshmallow – preferably ringing the changes.

If you suffer from intestinal gas, drink a litre a day of an infusion of bilberry leaves or blackberries, with wholewheat purée, rice or barley water (see p. 92), to which you add pectin or agar-agar. In any case, you must drink at least half a litre of fluid a day, either of water or some infusion.

Your only solid food should be cereal purée or gruel – linseed, oats, whole wheat – of which you may take 2–5 bowls daily.

2 Subsequently, until you are completely recovered you may add:

Fresh fruit and vegetable juices. If the heartburn has stopped, you can include orange and grapefruit juice. Mix all juices, especially at first, with 1 part of linseed or sesame gruel to 2 parts juice.

Dairy products: 2 or 3 yoghourts per day, plus 150g (5–6 oz) whey or fresh buttermilk.

Vegetable milk: almond milk, with 5–10 drops of lemon juice, but no sugar.

Other drinks: soothing infusions and non-sparkling mineral water.

For a quick recovery, eat nothing else while on this diet. If you are in real pain, put hot packs on your stomach and abdomen, to help you relax. Drink a camomile infusion after meals. If you have to travel, eat three or four almonds, chewing them slowly. Make sure you relax as much as possible.

Have a camomile enema each day (see the appendix on Types of Treatment) to rid your intestine of whatever has made you ill. Stay in bed if possible, and be sure to keep warm.

*Note:* This is the ideal diet for a young child with a digestive upset, or who is prone to digestive problems.

## HAEMORRHOIDS

It is hard to know quite why haemorrhoids, or piles, are so often treated as a joke, or why people find them embarrassing. They are merely varicose veins in an awkward place. The word 'haemorrhoid' comes from the Greek, and means 'veins liable to discharge blood'. They do in fact bleed at times, which usually brings a sensation of relief. They are painful, whether they are internal or external, and especially so when most distended. With Dr Bircher-Benner's treatment, relief is almost immediate.

1 Acute attacks are generally caused by constipation, which of course intensifies the pain. Treat it at once, therefore, with mild, vegetable-based laxatives and camomile enemas.

2 Sit in a very cold bath for 10 minutes two or three times a day. This reduces congestion.

3 Give up all meat, hot spices, condiments and alcohol.

Even a single grain of pepper or a small sip of wine will increase the congestion in the veins of the rectum and make them more painful.

Diet as follows:

1 For one to three days, a complete detoxication treatment to purify the system. Take only fruit and vegetable juices, and in the morning and evening a cup of witch-hazel tea (witch-hazel helps the circulation, having a liquefying and decongesting effect on the blood). Do not, however, expect instant results: any lapse in the treatment may cause the pain to recur.

2 To prevent any recurrence, stick to the following diet for three weeks:

Fresh fruit and vegetable juices

Vegetable milks

Vegetable bouillon and fresh vegetable soups

Cooked vegetables (any sort)

Meat: none until you are completely better. One small piece of beef could trigger another attack

Fish: non-oily fish, not more than once a week

Eggs: one or two per week

Fats: 15–20g (½–¾ oz) unsalted butter per day; pure olive or other cold-pressed oil

Dairy products: all except fermented cheese

Drinks: non-sparkling mineral water and herb teas; make sure you have 2 large cups of witch-hazel tea daily

Cereals: alone or in muesli. Avoid rice, as it has a constipating effect.

*Absolutely no* alcohol, chocolate, coffee or stimulants of any kind, or fried food.

## THE HEART

The blood vessels served by the heart are 100,000 kilometres long – two and a half times the circumference of the earth. The heart beats 40 million times a year and pumps 2,538,000 litres of blood. Nor can it ever stop for a moment. It does have a chance to slow down at night, yet we relentlessly make it work overtime, going out to dinners and parties, staying up late to watch television. Our hearts are made to last a hundred years but, as Dr Bircher-Benner used to say, we weaken them by smoking, we attack them with knives and forks. 'Of everyone who dies of heart failure it can be said that he smoked too much, ate too much, and rested too little.'

On its long journey, the blood has certain fuelling stations – for instance, the intestine, where it finds energy-giving substances such as vitamins, sugars and mineral salts. Yet day by day we provide it with poisonous substances, and people often have to pay in middle age for the excesses of youth. But if the cardiac muscle is not too damaged it can be repaired – contrary to popular belief that heart disease is incurable. Of course, only a doctor can *treat* heart disease, but the right diet and sensible precautions can prevent it, and can also provide valuable support for the medical treatment.

To prevent heart disease, then, give your heart a rest. It is largely a matter of common sense.

1 Adopt a regular rhythm of life.

2 At the first warning sign, go to bed and rest. At other times, make sure you get eight hours' sleep by going to bed early (the sleep before midnight is the most restorative).

3 Go for an early morning walk, but do not tire yourself out.

4 Have ten minutes a day of suitable gymnastic and breathing exercises.

5 Take an hour's rest in the middle of the day.

6 Make sure you get enough fresh air (air-bathing), warmth and sunshine. Stimulate your circulation with hydrotherapy – alternating foot baths, arm baths, alter-

nating showers, hot compresses, Priessnitz packs for the trunk. (See the appendix for all these.)

7 The intestine should be clear: if you are constipated, have a camomile enema every other day.

8 Your diet should exclude salt or irritants of any kind. *Remember:* obesity is enemy number one! If you are overweight, this is the very first problem you must deal with if you are not to put too much strain on your heart.

The following diet is the same for all heart problems:

(i) *The first two days:*
Stay in bed without eating, and drink a 200g (7 oz) glass of orange or grapefruit juice four times a day.

(ii) *For one week, drink daily*
   4 large glasses of fruit juice
   150g (5–6 oz) fresh vegetable juice
   150g (5–6 oz) almond milk
   2 150g (5–6 oz) glasses of buttermilk
   1 or 2 cups of rose-hip tea, or golden-rod tea if you are not urinating freely.
*Remember* that digestion makes demands on the heart and can tire it; you can rest it by having three or four small meals in a day instead of the usual two large ones.

(iii) *For the next few weeks, and until you are really better, a salt-free diet:*
   Morning:      Muesli and fruit
                 Wholemeal bread (without salt) and vegetable margarine
                 Rose-hip tea
   Midday:       Fresh fruit
                 Raw vegetables with dressing of sunflower oil and lemon juice (see table of suggestions, p. 84)
                 Vegetable bouillon
                 Cooked fresh vegetables, potatoes or cereals

*Evening:*            Muesli and fruit
                      Soup with wholemeal bread
                      Rose-hip tea
*During the day:* 150g (5–6 oz) vegetable milk (almond,
                      pine-kernel, sesame seed) and 300g
                      (10–11 oz) buttermilk, divided as
                      convenient.


## HIGH CHOLESTEROL LEVEL

Of all the various kinds of fats, the one we are most preoc-
cupied with today is cholesterol: it is found in large
amounts in the deposits that cause arteriosclerosis – the
disease responsible for over half of all deaths of people
over the age of 45. The outside source of excess cholesterol as such is animal food, and especially animal fats. As
with all illnesses caused by defective nutrition, Bircher-
Benner dietetic cures can work wonders.

1  For one week: a strict diet that will in most cases reduce cholesterol to a normal level.

Permitted foods:

Fresh fruit and vegetable juices: any

Fresh fruit: any

Raw and cooked vegetables: any, but as many green
leafy vegetables as possible.

Soups: some vegetable bouillon daily

Cereals: any – either in muesli or by themselves

Fats: wheatgerm oil, walnut oil, and above all sunflower oil, which prevents cholesterol build-up.

Dairy products: buttermilk (when it can be obtained),
yoghourt, and small quantities of skim milk

Sweetenings: honey and unrefined brown sugar

*Absolutely no* salt, hot spices, stimulants, tobacco, alcohol,
cakes, chocolate, sweets, animal fat.

2  Continue for the next few months with the following diet:

Fresh fruit and vegetable juices

Fresh and dried fruit

Vegetables, raw or cooked, with as many salads and raw vegetables as possible.

Soups

Cereal dishes, especially muesli

Fats: the same oils as on the strict diet (20 – 30g or ½ – 1½ oz per day) plus purées of walnuts, hazelnuts, almonds, sesame seed and soya

Dairy products: small amounts of raw milk, yoghourt, low-fat cheese, buttermilk

Sweetenings: unrefined brown sugar, honey

One or two eggs per week

Meat: once or twice a week if you feel you must

Non-oily fish: as meat

*Absolutely no* fried food, game, offal, rich sauces, salt, hot spices, tobacco, or alcohol

Remember, and this is important, that cholesterol is present only in animal foods (brains, offal, egg-yolk, butter, shellfish, whole milk – which contains 12mg of cholesterol per litre)

## HYPERTENSION

Hypertension (high blood pressure) or a high cholesterol level (and the two usually go together) must never be neglected. Hypertension leads to cardio-vascular disease, which kills even more people than road accidents do, causing up to 50 per cent of all adult deaths.

Diet is one of the major causes. Animal fats, as well as raising the cholesterol level, cause high blood pressure, and the meat we get today, from animals fed with hormones, constitutes an additional risk. Salt, too, should be cut out or kept to a minimum where there is any sign of hypertension.

If you suffer from breathlessness, palpitations, a sense of suffocation, and of increased tension, then unless you want to become a candidate for arterial disease you must make an immediate change in your way of life – and stick to it rigidly.

1 Rest: lead a regular life that is calm and, above all, quiet: noise is one of man's greatest enemies today. If you cannot get away from noise, at least have half an hour's rest in the middle of the day: this can be taken in your office, lying back in a chair with the curtains drawn or the blinds down. If your office is noisy, use wax ear-plugs. A good night's rest is also essential: if you have high blood pressure you must have the resolution to go to bed early.

2 Breathing: slow, deep breathing helps to lower the blood pressure. Spend a few minutes several times a day breathing slowly in and out; if you are tense or worried (also a factor in causing hypertension), this will help you to calm down.

3 Relaxation is vital. You must learn to lie down as though you were dead: relax all your muscles and empty your mind. Make sure you have twenty minutes' relaxation of this kind after work and before dinner.

4 Hydrotherapy helps restore the circulation: baths, and wet packs at night; as well as foot baths, sitting-baths, and brushing the skin (see the appendix) – all of which stimulate the circulation and relax the nerves and muscles.

5 A salt-free diet is a *must*. In other respects, the diet is as follows:

(i) *For 15 to 30 days:*
Fruit juices: any
Vegetable juices: any
Fresh fruit: any
Fresh vegetables: any. But with both fruit and vege-

tables, priority should be given to those containing vitamins B6, E, C, and niacin which help to lower the blood pressure (see Table of Vitamins)

Vegetable bouillon: some every day

Cereals: whole wheat and all cereals, but in small quantities if you are overweight

Meat: absolutely none

Fish: absolutely none

Fats: pure olive or other cold-pressed oil; not more than 30g (1 oz) butter a day

Dairy products: buttermilk, whey, yoghourt, low-fat soft cheese

Eggs: one or two per week

Sweetening: a very little unrefined brown sugar or pure honey

*Absolutely no* hot spices, or stimulants (no tobacco, wine, spirits, coffee or tea).

*Note*: If you also have a high cholesterol level, this diet should be replaced by the anti-cholesterol crash diet (p. 138).

(ii) *For several months, you should stick to the following diet:*

Fruit juices: any

Vegetable juices: any

Fresh and dried fruit and nuts: any; almonds, walnuts and hazelnuts should be eaten every day, but in very small quantities

Vegetable bouillon: some every day

Cereals: any, but in moderation if you are overweight or tend to become so; one or two slices of wholemeal bread

Meat: only if you feel you cannot do without it; 120g (4–5 oz) of beef may be eaten, grilled, every other day

Fish: small helpings of freshwater fish only

Fats: pure olive or other unsaturated oil; not more than 30g (1 oz) butter per day

Dairy products: buttermilk, whey, yoghourt, low-fat soft cheese

Eggs: one or two per week

Sweetening: small amounts of unrefined brown sugar or pure honey

*Absolutely no* hot spices, or stimulants (tobacco, wine, spirits, coffee, tea).

## INSOMNIA

Insomnia is not an illness, though lack of sleep can result in quite serious mental disturbance. If you go to your doctor complaining that you 'can't sleep a wink at night', he is all too likely to give you sleeping pills. Then it will not be long before you have to take larger doses in order to get a heavy, dreamless, unrestful night, which leaves you knocked out the next morning and needing amphetamines to keep you going. This vicious circle can lead to serious depression and the consulting-room of the neurologist or psychiatrist.

What causes insomnia? It can be a sedentary life, and eating rich food in the evening. It can also be persistent mental stress: worries and annoyances that keep your mind alert and prevent your sleeping, even though you feel exhausted. In neither case will you be helped by drugs.

But it is important to realise that not everyone needs the same amount of sleep, nor does the same person necessarily need the same amount at different ages. There is no point in being determined to get your eight hours if your body is in fact only asking for seven, or six, or even less. Dr Bircher-Benner, as we have seen, managed to cure his insomnia with Priessnitz packs, and prescribed them to patients, telling them to go to bed at eight, so as to benefit from the 'hours before midnight'. He also recommended that, should they wake in the middle of the night, even at 3 a.m., they should go for a short walk, after which they would sleep very well.

Some people who cannot sleep may merely be lacking vitamin B6, the 'sleep vitamin'. If so, they can get it from wholemeal bread, pumpernickel bread, blackstrap molasses, and green vegetables. If calcium is lacking, a glass of milk before bed will help.

A cup of lime-flower tea, flavoured with one or two spoonfuls of orange-flower water, or a cup of orange-flower tea, may help you to sleep, too, but in cases of serious insomnia, the Priessnitz pack (see appendix) is the only thing that works.

## THE LIVER

Everyone must have had a 'bilious attack' at some time. Digestive upsets, a coated tongue, sallow complexion, nausea, vomiting, flatulence, depression have all been ascribed, rightly or wrongly, to the liver. What is quite certain is that our denatured food does not give the liver the nutrients it needs, whereas a Bircher-Benner diet does.

The liver also reacts to worry and nervous tension, which can affect it as much as physical causes. But, as Dr Bircher-Benner warned, 'liverish' symptoms can mean something more serious; they can be the warning signs of a more complicated illness – jaundice or hepatitis – or an indication that the liver has become 'worn out before its time' by continuous ill treatment. So do not attempt to make your own diagnosis. It is vital to consult your doctor, who will make the necessary tests to find out what is wrong.

In cases of ordinary 'biliousness', here is the Bircher-Benner treatment.

1 Try to live as regular a life as possible.

2 Get eight hours' sleep at night, and rest for twenty minutes after lunch.

3 Take at least two short walks a day – one when you get up in the morning and one before you go to bed.

4 Take a tepid shower every day (not cold, which would be a shock to the liver). In summer, wrap yourself in wet packs (especially during an attack).

5 Exercise is good providing it is not too tiring – swimming, golf, or walking, for example.

6 Try to have holidays, however short, at regular intervals. A week every two or three months is the ideal, but even a weekend in the country makes a good break.

7 Try to avoid worry, argument, things that make you angry or tense. (Make it clear to those around you that keeping calm is part of the treatment.)

8 Finally, help your liver by giving up food that upsets it; this will vary from one person to another – it could be eggs, butter, oil, cream, chocolate – and you simply have to find out for yourself.

The dietary part of the treatment is as follows:

(i) *One day of fasting*, on which you have only bitter tea (see p. 109), fruit juices with some lemon in them, and plenty of infusions. On the evening of that day have a hot foot-bath, then make yourself a Priessnitz pack (see the appendix) and go to bed early.

(ii) *For the next few weeks, follow the diet set out below.* In addition, if you are in pain, a cup of thyme tea will bring relief. Apply a hot compress to your liver each day, and lie down for half an hour.

**Diet**

Raw vegetable juices with a few drops of lemon: carrot, radish, sauerkraut, dandelion

Fresh fruit: especially thin slices of apple

Raw vegetables: grated and dressed with lemon juice and a little buttermilk: carrots, radishes, globe artichokes (very good for the liver)

Cooked vegetables: all vegetables in season except cabbage; mashed potatoes with a little buttermilk

Soups: vegetable bouillon (with no fat)

Cereals: whole grains, ground or flaked, by themselves or in soup (without fat), muesli or wholemeal bread (in small amounts)

Dairy products: low-fat soft cheese, low-fat yoghourt, buttermilk (as much as you like)

Drinks: Infusions: – peppermint tea, gentian tea, bitter tea, aniseed tea (3–4 cups a day). Mineral water as advised by the doctor

Sweetening: only pure honey

*Absolutely no* fats (butter, cream, oil), eggs, chocolate, condiments (pepper, mustard), or stimulants (alcohol, coffee, tobacco).

(iii) *For a month after all symptoms have disappeared, your diet may be extended to include*

Dried fruit: raisins, dried figs

Fats: unsalted butter (not more than 20g (1 oz) per day), pure olive oil. The butter should never be cooked or mixed with the oil

Vegetable milks: all

Meat: if you feel you cannot do without it you may have grilled meat once a week towards the end of your diet

Fish: as meat – but non-oily fish only

*Avoid*: cream, milk, walnuts, white bread, white flour and sugar, sauces, eggs, meat and oily fish.

*Absolutely no*: alcohol, coffee, melted fats, offal, fried food, pastries, or cakes, chocolate, fat cheeses, mayonnaise, ice or iced drinks.

*Note*: It is important to ensure that your intestine is clear.

In case of constipation, have a camomile enema (see the appendix on Types of Treatment).

## OBESITY

Obesity is an unattractive condition: it is also dangerous. It leads to a gradual deterioration of the organism, affecting the whole of the bone and ligament structure, causing distortion of the legs, and making arthritis more likely. It may also be the cause of certain kinds of diabetes, and is a major factor in arteriosclerosis, hypertension and cardio-vascular disease. The fat do not only find life uncomfortable – they find it shorter. Life expectation may be reduced by from eight to ten years for the seriously overweight.

It is high time, therefore, to dispel the myth of the 'bonny' baby, or the jovial fat man who lives well. However little you may think you eat, if you are overweight you must be eating more than you need. Rare indeed is the obesity due to hormone imbalance or other specific illness. In the vast majority of cases, diet alone is responsible. The reasons for overeating vary enormously, though, and Dr Bircher-Benner always spent a long time examining obese patients.

The roots of this problem are diverse and they go very deep. People seldom eat too much because they are hungry: the fevered voracity of the fat usually conceals some underlying problem. Overeating is a refuge for the lonely, the depressed, the shy; it comforts the 'unloved'. The classic case is the woman who puts on weight because she has lost her husband – or given up trying to find one. The lack of willpower that makes it impossible to stick to a diet generally has a profound psychological basis.

There is unfortunately no miracle cure for obesity, and the only hope of losing weight is to stop believing that there is one. Most people have taken years to accumulate the excess, and they must realise that it will take months to lose. However, the Bircher-Benner slimming cure – known at the clinic as the 'cure de sveltesse' – is miraculous to the extent that the weight lost is lost for good, for the patient comes to adopt a whole new way of eating. You may find it surprising that the diet is so precise, specifying 'six walnuts, four almonds', and so on. The point is that it is a perfecty balanced diet, and these quantities represent the amount of energy that is needed. It must therefore be very strictly followed.

**Some general rules**
Throughout the diet, drink two or three glasses of golden-rod infusion (as a diuretic, see p. 109) over the course of each day, and a cup (150g – 5–6 oz) of rose-hip tea at every meal after the first day.

Where lemon juice is specified, this should not be more than the juice of half a lemon.

Salads and raw vegetables may be mixed with a very small amount of olive or sunflower oil, 10g (½ oz) per day. No salt or spices.

If you are constipated, take camomile enemas, one or two spoonfuls of psyllium seeds or some boldo-leaf tea.

Rest is important: have an hour's rest after lunch, and go to bed early. Go for a half-hour walk morning and evening. Sunbathing is excellent, but not for more than an hour at a time. Alternating showers should be taken (see the appendix on Types of Treatment).
*Absolutely no* wine, spirits or stimulants.

*First week*
 *First day* (fasting – if staying in bed)
  *Morning:* 200g (7 oz) orange and lemon juice, or other
      fresh fruit juice

*Midday:*    200g (7 oz) carrot, celery and lemon juice, or
other vegetable juice
*Evening:*   200g (7 oz.) orange juice

*First day* (fasting – if *not* staying in bed)
*Morning:* 200g (7 oz) orange and grapefruit juice
*Midday:*    100g (3–4 oz) yoghourt (no sugar)
200g (7 oz) tomato, spinach and celery juice
150g (5–6 oz) vegetable bouillon
*Afternoon:* 200g (7 oz) orange juice
*Evening:*   200g (7 oz) carrot and lemon juice
150g (5–6 oz) yoghourt

*Second day*
*Morning:* 150g (5–6 oz) orange juice or muesli
150g (5–6 oz) yoghourt
*Midday:*    1 apple, pear or other fruit
200–250g (7–9 oz) raw vegetables: cabbage
(with cumin), celery, green pepper (with
shallots)
200g (7 oz) cooked vegetables: e.g. leeks
1 baked potato (80–100g; 3–4 oz) with
sesame seeds
*Evening:*   180g (6–7 oz) muesli with 10g (½ oz) grated
nuts
150g (5–6 oz) celery bouillon with parsley
1 slice wholemeal bread
50g (2 oz) low-fat soft cheese (with chives)

*Third day*
*Morning:* 150g (5–6 oz) mandarin and lemon juice
1 wholemeal crispbread
150g (5–6 oz) yoghourt
*Midday:*    1 apple, 1 orange, 6 grapes
200–250g (7–9 oz) raw vegetables: lamb's
lettuce, beetroot, parsley, black radishes,
celery
150g (5–6 oz) vegetable bouillon

6 walnuts, 4 almonds
*Evening:* 1 pear, 1 apple and 250g (9 oz) muesli
50g (2 oz) low-fat soft cheese (with cumin)

*Fourth day*
*Morning:* 150g (5–6 oz) orange juice with lemon
150g (5–6 oz) muesli
1 wholemeal crispbread
*Midday:* 1 apple, 1 orange, 1 dried fig
200–250g (7–9 oz) raw vegetables: lettuce or
watercress salad, tomato (with rosemary or
basil), raw sauerkraut (with juniper berries),
radishes
200g (7 oz) cooked vegetables: courgettes,
spinach
Brown rice (4 tablespoons)
*Evening:* 150g (5–6 oz) muesli
150g (5–6 oz) vegetable bouillon
1 slice wholemeal bread
50g (2 oz) low-fat soft cheese (with chives)

*Fifth day* (day of rest)
*Morning:* 200g (7 oz) orange juice with lemon
*Midday:* 200g (7 oz) mandarin juice
200g (7 oz) spinach, carrot, celery juice
150g (5–6 oz) yoghourt
*Evening:* 200g (7 oz) grapefruit juice
150g (5–6 oz) vegetable bouillon
150g (5–6 oz) yoghourt

*Sixth day*
*Morning:* 180g (6–7 oz) muesli
1 wholemeal crispbread
*Midday:* 1 apple, 1 orange
200–250g (7–9 oz) raw vegetables: lettuce,
globe artichoke with olive oil, black radishes
(with cumin),

           cucumber with yoghourt dressing
*Evening:*  1 pear
           180g (6–7 oz) muesli with 10g (½ oz) grated
           nuts
           2 wholemeal crispbreads
           6 walnuts, 4 almonds, 6 hazelnuts
           50g (2 oz) low-fat soft cheese (with cumin)

## Seventh day

*Morning:*  200g (7 oz) oranges with lemon juice, or
           muesli
           2 wholemeal crispbreads
           100g (3–4 oz) yoghourt
*Midday:*  1 pear, 1 apple, 10 grapes
           200–250g (7–9 oz) raw vegetables: green
           salad: tomato (with parsley), celery, white
           cabbage (with cumin)
           4 tablespoonfuls mashed potato
*Evening:*  180g (6–7 oz) muesli
           150g (5–6 oz) vegetable soup
           2 slices wholemeal bread
           50g (2 oz) low-fat soft cheese

## Second week

*First day* – fruit only
  *Morning:*  250g (9 oz) of whatever fruit you like, plus 1
               apple, 1 orange
  *Midday:*  250g (9 oz) fruit, plus 1 banana, 1 mandarin
  *Evening:*  250g (9 oz) fruit, plus 1 apple, 1 pear

*Second and third days*
As second and third days of first week

*Fourth day* – semi-fasting
  *Morning:*  250g (9 oz) orange juice
               150g (5–6 oz) yoghourt

| | |
|---|---|
| *Midday:* | 1 orange, 1 banana |
| | 1 dried fig or a few raisins |
| *Evening:* | 1 apple |
| | 150g (5–6 oz) vegetable bouillon |

The fifth, sixth and seventh days as the fifth, sixth and seventh days of the first week.

### Third week
No fasting this week. Repeat the diets of the second, fourth and seventh days of the first week throughout the week.

### Fourth week
Start this week with one day's fasting on fruit juices only; then repeat diets of the second, fourth and seventh day of the first week for the remaining days.

If you have not lost enough weight over these four weeks, the following diet may be continued until you have (quantities as for the preceding diet):

| | |
|---|---|
| *Morning:* | fruit |
| | Muesli or 2 slices wholemeal bread with butter |
| | Rose-hip tea |
| *Midday:* | Fruit |
| | Raw vegetables |
| | 2 cooked vegetables |
| | Soup or dessert |
| | Rose-hip tea |
| *Evening:* | Fruit |
| | Muesli |
| | Low-fat cheese |
| | Rose-hip tea |

Avoid too much fat (30g (1 oz) maximum per day) and

protein, and do not exceed 1,200 calories a day. Once a week, on Sunday perhaps, have a day's rest (staying in bed and fasting on fruit and vegetable juices only).

For a year after this, you can plan your diet as follows:
1 Once a month, preferably at a weekend or on a non-working day, plan a fruit day.

> *Morning:* 250g (9 oz) of whatever fruit you like, plus 1
> apple, 1 orange
> *Midday:* 250g (9 oz) fruit, plus 1 banana, 1 mandarin
> *Evening:* 250g (9 oz) fruit, plus 1 apple, 1 pear

2 After three months, repeat the first week of the diet.
3 After six months, repeat the first two weeks of the diet.
4 After a year, repeat the first three weeks of the diet.

## THE SKIN

Helena Rubinstein used to come to the Bircher-Benner clinic for a cure every year until she died – at the age of ninety. The first time she came, in about 1935, she was so struck by the beautiful skin of the clinic nurses that she was convinced, despite their denials, that they must be using some wonderful, mystery beauty cream that was more effective than any of her own products. They assured her over and over again that their only beauty treatment was their diet, and when she finally realised that this was true she started sending clients she had failed to help to the clinic for the same treatment. Time and again, they would return home with complexions like young children.

Madame Rubinstein was so impressed that she wanted Dr Bircher-Benner to go into business with her. In her view, science should be placed at the service of commerce, and she was astounded when he refused her offer. Undeterred, however, she launched the Bircher-Benner cure herself in her New York salons, christening it 'A Day for Beauty'.

Dull or peeling skin, pimples and blackheads are all symptoms of malnutrition and of an unhealthy life without enough sunshine and fresh air. We are inclined to forget that the skin is an organ of elimination: it rids the blood of poisons, but when these become excessive the skin cannot cope with them and becomes clogged up. Everyone whose skin is oily or dry and lifeless needs a treatment to cleanse the whole system (see Detoxication, p. 127), plus additional vitamin C (lemons, oranges, carrots, green vegetables – see Vitamin Table), and a diet in which animal protein is replaced by vegetable.

Note especially that tobacco is your skin's worst enemy. If women realised the damage cigarettes do to their complexions, even the least vain would give up smoking.

Whether your skin is dry or oily, the Bircher treatment is as follows:

The day before you start your treatment, take a vegetable laxative. Then:

1 *One or two days' complete fasting (in bed if possible) with only fruit and vegetable juices:*

    *Morning:*  200g (7 oz) fruit juice, according to season
                150g (5–6 oz) almond milk
                1 cup rose-hip tea
    *Midday:*  200g (7 oz) fruit juice
                150g (5–6 oz) vegetable juice
                150g (5–6 oz) soya milk
    *Evening:*  as morning

2 *Then for one week:*

    *Morning:*  250g (9 oz) muesli with fruit according to season
                150g (5–6 oz) fruit, according to season
                1 cup of golden-rod tea (as a diuretic)

*Midday:*    150g (5–6 oz) fresh fruit, and 20g (¾ oz)
            dried fruit or nuts (not peanuts)
            Raw vegetables without seasoning
*Evening:* As morning
3 *For the next week:*
*Morning:* Muesli
            150g (5–6 oz) fruit, according to season
            Wholemeal bread with walnut butter or
            vegetable margarine
            Herb tea (whichever flavour you prefer)
*Midday:*   Raw fruit
            Raw vegetables according to season, with
            seasoning
            Cooked vegetables with a little vegetable
            margarine
*Evening:* As morning
4 *Then continue as follows, until the skin is completely clear,*
*with no pimples or blackheads:*
*Morning:* Muesli
            Fruit
            Wholemeal bread with butter
            Herb tea
*Midday:*   Fruit
            Raw vegetables
            Cooked dishes – vegetables, pasta, rice
*Evening:* Muesli or fruit salad
            Yoghourt
            Wholemeal bread and vegetable margarine
            Low-fat cheese
Fruit should always be eaten at the *beginning* of the meal
and in the quantities recommended above.

In addition to diet, the following external treatment
should be followed:

Sunbathing: start with 5 minutes at a time and increase
gradually to 1 hour – never more. In winter, this may be
replaced by using a sun-lamp, but only under medical
supervision.

Air-bathing (see the appendix on Types of Treatment),
daily walks
Alternating showers, hot and cold (see appendix)

The treatment normally takes three months, but when the
skin is badly affected, it may be some time before it is
completely recovered.

It is advisable to keep in good condition by taking an
'overhaul' cure for a month out of every year.

## VARICOSE VEINS

Women tend to blame pregnancy for their varicose veins,
but they are often wrong to do so. Varicose veins do not
appear out of the blue – they develop where there has
been earlier weakness. The time to look at your veins is
when you are twenty. If you see little clusters of tiny
bluish-red veins round your ankles or knees, you should
take action at once. You must introduce a new discipline
into your life, watching your weight and your diet. Albumin and cholesterol become attached to the walls of the
veins and impair their elasticity. You must also make yourself take exercise: walking, running and swimming exert
muscular pressure on the veins which keeps the blood
moving at a good pace.

If you only discover the problem when the damage is
already done, then following Dr Bircher-Benner's treatment will prevent the development of more serious conditions such as varicose ulcers, or even phlebitis.

1 For three days you must undergo a detoxication cure
to cleanse the system, taking only fruit and vegetable juices
and diuretic infusions.

2 For at least a month, observe the following diet:
Fresh fruit juices: any
Fresh vegetable juices: any

Vegetable milks: almond, etc.

Witch-hazel tea

Soups: fresh vegetable soups, and vegetable bouillon

Cooked vegetables: any

Cereals: any, wholemeal bread, muesli

Meat: not more than once a week, and never when veins are painful

Fish: as meat

Eggs: 1 or 2 per week

Fats: fresh butter (10–15g (⅓–½ oz) per day), pure olive or other vegetable oil

Dairy products: milk, cheese (gruyère type and soft, slightly salted cheese), cottage cheese, sour milk, skim milk

Sweetening: unrefined sugar, honey, molasses

Decaffeinated coffee occasionally

Salt: as your doctor advises

*Absolutely no* wine, spirits, beer, aperitifs, cocoa

Meanwhile, you should also be doing the following:

Resting: lie down several times a day (if only for 10 minutes) with feet and legs higher than your head, to stimulate circulation. Sleep in the same position at night.

Sunbathing: do this in the early morning or late afternoon when the sun is not so hot that it dilates your veins rather than making them supple.

*Caution:* Do not sunbathe if your blood pressure is high.

Take a cold shower immediately after sunbathing; when there is no sun, warm up in a hot shower first, and then have a cold one. Also take alternating foot-baths (see appendix on Types of Treatment).

Some walking and exercises. When you are at home, or on the beach, go barefoot. And remember that swimming is the best form of exercise for the legs.

# Appendices

# Types of Treatment

### Agar-agar
A colourless jelly extracted from certain algae. Used in jellies and jams, and may be added to juices. Excellent for constipation, because it facilitates passage through the intestine.

### Algae
Cryptogamic plants living on the sea-bed. They have many uses. Edible algae differ from non-edible in that they have a greater content of mineral salts, and bromine (a simple metalloid substance that acts as a revealing agent: sodium bromide, potassium bromide, magnesium bromide).

### Air-bathing
Very good for the circulation, the skin, and cardiac troubles. One should lie down in the shade, in a bathing suit, or, if possible, in the nude, for five minutes. The time can be gradually extended. Obviously this is only suitable on warm or hot days, and sheltered from the wind.

### Baths
*algae*: Follow the directions on the packet.

*alternating*: These are very good for cardiac troubles, but can usually only be taken in clinics, because two bath-tubs are needed. At home, you can achieve a similar effect with alternating showers (see below).

*for the arms*: Calming, very good for the heart, and for easing congestion in the head and the lungs. Especially useful for angina, since they help to dilate the arteries of the heart.

Plunge the arms up to above the elbows in water heated to 38°C (100°F). Add hot water until the temperature is 45°C (113°F). Keep them there for 20 minutes. Then rest in bed for from half an hour to an hour.

*for the feet*: Alternating foot-baths are soothing; they relieve headaches and help to cure insomnia.

Have two basins, one of hot water (45°C, 113°F), the other of cold. Immerse the feet in the hot water for 3 minutes and in the cold for 30 seconds. Repeat twice, ending with cold water.

*mud*: Excellent for rheumatism, arthritis, arthrosis. The best mud-baths are volcanic in origin. They are used mainly as part of a clinic cure, but one can sometimes buy mud preparations from pharmacists, and this, though not as effective as fresh mud, has often been successful.

*sand*: Excellent for arthritis in the hands. Heat some dry, fine sand to a temperature of about 40°C (104°F), plunge the hands into it, and move them about.

*sedative baths*: These relieve tension and insomnia. The bath should be at a temperature of 37–38°C (98–100°F), and you can remain in it for up to an hour (10 minutes is the minimum). The longer the time, the more soothing is the effect, but continue adding hot water to keep the temperature constant.

Try a pine-needle bath – include a large spoonful of pine needles in a bath. An alternative is a lime-flower bath: here, you infuse 500g (1 lb) lime flowers in a litre of water, and add to a hot bath. This latter is especially good for children.

*sitting baths*: Hay-flower baths are helpful for gynaecological and intestinal pain; they ease the bladder and assist urination, and also help to bring on menstruation. Oak-bark baths relieve congestion of the bladder in cases of cystitis.

Add 250g (about ½ lb) of one or other to the water in a hip-bath or ordinary tub; the temperature of a hay-flower bath should be about 38°C (100°F), that of an oak-bark bath 35–43°C (95–108°F). Stay in the bath for 15–20 minutes.

**Brushing**
This activates the circulation and is very good for the skin. Use a semi-hard brush (never nylon) and brush each part of the body in turn. This should take from 5 to 10 minutes.

**Clay**
Clay is the pure natural form of aluminium silicate. It is used in medicine (after sterilisation) because it contains in the natural state all the mineral salts necessary for life. It is extremely effec-

tive in all deficiency diseases and has a beneficial effect on the body. A prime example of a natural medicament.

A clay compress – made by mixing clay with water to the consistency of a thick paste — can be applied locally to ease pain in severe arthritic attacks.

### Compresses

*cold*: Good for any illness where there is enlargement of the heart or risk of stasis of the blood. Makes breathing easier. Apply for 30 minutes not more than three times a day.

*hot*: Helps to dilate the coronary arteries. Extremely good for cardiac cases and patients suffering from angina.

Hot compresses may be wet or dry. If wet, they must be reasonably thick, and must be renewed before they cool down. Alcohol compresses can be used in place of water. An ordinary hot-water bottle makes a perfectly good dry compress.

### Douches

*Kneipp douches*: Specially recommended to those with poor circulation, varicose veins or even ulcers.

The top of the body should remain covered for warmth, while the lower part is sprayed vigorously. The water should be tepid at first, and gradually allowed to become completely cold. Start with the feet, and work slowly up the legs to the thighs. Make sure the patient's feet are warm before beginning the treatment.

The arms, shoulders and back may be treated in the same way.

*thigh douches*: Very good for the circulation; draws the blood down to the lower part of the body.

With as powerful a spray as possible, douche only the thighs and hips for 5 minutes with very hot water, then for 1 minute with cold. Breathe deeply, then repeat two or three times, ending with cold water.

### Enemas

In cases of constipation, a camomile enema may be used. A small handful of camomile flowers should be added to a litre of boiling water. Strain and use while still warm.

### Friction

Friction activates the circulation and is very good for the skin.

Rub each part of the body in turn, first with a towel wrung out in very hot water, then with another wrung out in cold. Finish off by rubbing down with a dry towel.

### Laxatives

*Linseed* is an excellent laxative. Wash 1 tablespoonful of linseed; cook for 10 minutes in 200 c.c. (⅓ pint) of water, strain and cool. This may be added to fruit or vegetable juice. Ground into flour, it is also useful for poultices. It can be bought in health-food shops; or, for external use only, from pharmacists.

*Psyllium seeds*: Soak 2 teaspoonfuls of seeds in tepid water for half an hour, then swallow with a little water. Best taken before going to bed at night.

### Priessnitz packs

Wonderfully soothing in cases of insomnia and high fever.

Start by making the patient very warm – either by sunbathing in the summer, or with a hot bath. Soak a sheet in cold water; wring it out thoroughly, and wrap the patient up in it like a mummy. Place a woollen blanket on the bed and, with the patient lying on it, wrap it completely round the cold sheet. Add another blanket. Within a short time, the patient will feel a gentle warmth.

It is best to apply this treatment in the evening, because it will enable the patient to sleep very well.

The same treatment can be given applying the cold sheet to the trunk only, from the armpits to the tops of the thighs.

### Showers, alternating

These stimulate the circulation and the skin.

Have the shower very warm for 2 minutes, then cold for half a minute. Continue to alternate in this way until the skin is red and you feel warm. Finish with a cold shower.

This is very good for people with cardiac problems, but in this case the warm shower should last for 10 minutes and the cold only 20–40 seconds.

**Sponging**
Patients with a high temperature should be sponged down rapidly with cold water, several times a day if necessary. This removes the nitrogenous waste and the salt eliminated by perspiration.

Alternating hot and cold water sponging is very good for patients with kidney complaints who have to stay in bed.

**Sunbathing**
Good for the skin and for general vitality; helps the body to absorb vitamin D.

Start with 5 minutes lying on the back, then 5 minutes on the stomach. Gradually increase to half an hour on each side. Follow with a cold shower.

Those with cardiac troubles are usually prescribed air-bathing instead.

**Sun-lamp treatment**
This must never be undertaken except under professional supervision, because of the risk of burning. It is decontractant, and very good for the skin providing it is carefully timed. The patient may be wrapped in a towel or sheet, to assist sweating. Follow with cold water friction and an hour's rest.

# Table of
# Daily Vitamin Requirements

| Vitamin | Sources | Requirement/day | |
|---------|---------|-----------------|--|
| A | Liver, fish oils, eggs, milk, butter, enriched margarine, carrots, green leafy vegetables | 750 mg | Toxic in excess as stored in the liver. Not destroyed by cooking |
| D | Fatty fish, fish oils, eggs, butter, enriched margarine | 2.5 mg | Also made by the action of sunlight on the skin |
| E | Vegetable oils | 15 mg | Increased requirement if large amounts of unsaturated fatty acids are eaten |
| K | Green vegetables | Not known | Made by bacteria in intestine |
| C | Fruit, especially citrus, green vegetables, potatoes | 30 mg | Destroyed by cooking |
| *B Complex* B$_1$ Thiamin | Yeast, liver, pork, whole-grain cereals | 1.5 mg | Requirement: increase with increase in carbohydrate intake |
| B$_2$ Riboflavin | Milk, yeast, meat, whole-grain cereals | 1.7 mg | |
| Nicotinic acid (Niacin) | Liver, meat, nuts, legumes, yeast, whole-grain cereals | 17 mg | Can also be made from the amino-acid tryptophan in the body |

| Vitamin | Sources | Requirement/day | |
|---|---|---|---|
| B6 Pyridoxine | Most foods | 2 mg | |
| Folic acid | Liver, green vegetables, yeast | 400 mg | Increased requirement in pregnancy. Deficiency results in anaemia |
| B12 | Animal products | 4 mg | |
| Pantothenic acid | Most foods | 10 mg | |
| Biotin | | Low | Made by intestinal bacteria |

*Notes on Vitamin Table*

Green vegetables appear to provide few proteins, but the biological value of those proteins is very high. Whole-grain cereal protein in combination with green vegetable protein in a proportion of 9 to 1 ensures unusual biological qualities. Milk protein in combination with potatoes is equally excellent.

Remember that whole-grain flours and flakes are to be specially recommended for their high vitamin content, which decreases with refining. A teaspoonful of wheatgerm can be taken daily as a tonic.

All milk products are rich in calcium and phosphorus, especially calcium; all therefore counter decalcification.

Almonds, peanuts, and walnuts are particularly high in protein. (Remember that calories are provided both by sugars and fats: dried fruit calories come from sugar, nut calories from fat.)

Meat, fish and eggs are all rich in phosphorus, but this, coupled with their deficiency of calcium, makes them acid-producing. Meat and fish should therefore be taken in combination with milk products, vegetables and fruits (all alkali-producing) to balance the diet.
    Meat and fish are essentially a source of protein, iron and the B vitamins, especially B2. Any diet with little or no meat should therefore contain plenty of whole-grain cereals to provide vitamins B1 and B2, and protein. (See Table of Calorie Equivalents.)

# Table of Calorie Equivalents

100g (3½ oz) meat
is equivalent to
¼ litre (8–9 oz) milk
is equivalent to

2 eggs
½ litre (18 oz) milk
125g (4–5 oz) sour milk
60g (2 oz) creamy gruyère cheese
2 small potatoes (250g – 9 oz)
  yoghourt
4 (120g – 4½ oz) petits suisses
  cheese

100g (3½ oz) butter
is equivalent to
100g (3½ oz) bread
is equivalent to

85g (3 oz) oil
100g (3½ oz) margarine
70g (2½ oz) wholemeal flour,
  porridge oats, or pasta
75g (2–3 oz) rice
350g (¾ lb) potatoes
90g (3 oz) dried fruit and nuts

# Bibliography

Books by Dr Max Bircher-Benner available in English:

*Children's Diet* (C.W. Daniel, London 1946)
*Fruit Dishes and Raw Vegetables* (C.W. Daniel, London 1951)
*Prevention of Incurable Disease* (J. Clarke, Cambridge 1959)
*Nutrition Plan for High Blood-Pressure Problems* (Pyramid Books, New York 1977)
*Nutrition Plan for Liver and Gall Bladder Problems* (Pyramid Books, New York 1977)

By Ruth Bircher, edited by Claire Loewenfeld:
*Eating Your Way to Health* (Faber, London 1961)

Other books by Dr Max Bircher-Benner are available in French from Editions Victor Attinger S.A., Ch. Neuchâtel, Switzerland.